WHO/SDE/PHE/FOS/99.1

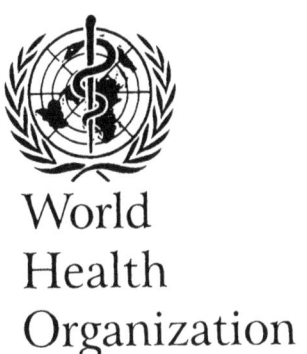

Geneva 1999

World Health Organization

Basic Food Safety for Health Workers

Dr Martin Adams

*School of Biological Sciences
University of Surrey, United Kingdom*

and

Dr Yasmine Motarjemi

*Food Safety Programme
Department of Protection of the Human Environment
World Health Organization, Switzerland*

This document has been prepared with the financial support of
Opec Fund for International Development
Vienna, Austria

World Health Organization
Geneva, Switzerland

© World Health Organization, 1999

This document is not a formal publication of the World Health Organization (WHO), and all rights are reserved by the Organization. The document may, however, be freely reviewed, abstracted, reproduced and translated, in part or in whole, but not for sale nor for use in conjunction with commercial purposes.

The views expressed in documents by named authors are solely the responsibility of those authors.

Contents

Acknowledgements 1
Introduction 3

Chapter 1

Foodborne illness 5

    Food in health and disease 5
    Extent of foodborne illness 8
    Foodborne illness: its definition and nature 10
        Infection 11
        Intoxication 11
    Infectious dose 12
    Health consequences of foodborne illness 13
    Economic impact of foodborne illness 16

Chapter 2

Foodborne hazards 17

    Biological hazards 17
        Parasites 17
        Viruses 18
        Bacteria 18
    Chemical hazards 18
        Industrial pollution of the environment 20
        Agricultural practices 21
        Food processing 22
        Natural toxicants in foods 23
        Biological sources 24
            Mycotoxins 24
            Algal toxins 26
    Physical hazards 27

Chapter 3

Factors leading to microbial foodborne illness 29

    Contamination - how do microorganisms get into food? 29
        Microorganisms that occur naturally in foods (indigenous microflora) 30
        Natural inhabitants of the environment 30
        Polluted environment: insanitary practices in agriculture and aquaculture 31
        Water 32
        Pests and pets 32
        The food handler 32
        Equipment, utensils and kitchen practices 33
    Growth 34
        Availability of nutrients 35
        Temperature 35
        Acidity/pH 36
        Water activity (a_w) 37
        Oxygen (air) 38
        Antimicrobial agents 38
        Time 38
    Survival 39
        Major factors leading to foodborne illness 41

Chapter 4

Hazards associated with different foods and their control 43

    Red meat, poultry and their products 43
    Eggs and egg products 45
    Milk and dairy products 45
    Fish, shellfish and fishery products 46
    Fruits and vegetables 49
    Cereals and cereal products 51
    Bottled waters 51

Chapter 5

Technologies for the control of hazards 53

    Technologies that prevent contamination 53
        Packaging 53
        Cleaning and disinfection of equipment and utensils 54
        Hygienic design of equipment 55
    Technologies that control microbial growth 55
    Technologies that remove or kill microorganisms in food 56
        Heat treatment 56
        Canned foods 57
        UHT processing/aseptic packaging 58
        Ionizing irradiation 59
        Ultraviolet irradiation 59
        Washing and disinfection 59

Chapter 6

Hygiene in food preparation 61

- Physical factors: premises and equipment 62
- Operational factors: hygienic handling of food 63
- Personal factors: personal hygiene and training 64
- The Hazard Analysis and Critical Control Point (HACCP) system 65

Chapter 7

The role of health workers in food safety 69

- The curative role 69
- The preventive role: controlling foodborne hazards 69
  - *Domestic food handlers* 70
    - Expectant mothers 70
    - Lactating women 70
    - Mothers of older infants and young children 71
  - *Professional food handlers* 71
  - *High-risk groups and people preparing food for them* 71
    - Travellers 71
    - The elderly 71
    - The sick 72
    - The undernourished 72
  - *The community* 72
    - Refugees 72
    - Schoolchildren 72
    - Street food vendors and food service establishments 73
- Surveillance 73

References 75

Bibliography 77

Appendix 1
Causative agents of foodborne illness 79

Appendix 2
WHO's Ten Golden Rules for Safe Food Preparation 113

Appendix 3
The Hazard Analysis and Critical Control Point System (HACCP) 115

Acknowledgements

Basic Food Safety for Health Workers has been prepared with a view to strengthening the education and training of health professionals in food safety. The book has been prepared by Drs Martin Adams, School of Biological Sciences, University of Surrey, United Kingdom and Yasmine Motarjemi, Food Safety Programme, World Health Organization. The contribution of Mrs Ann Dale, Mrs Francoise Fontannaz, Annette Enevoldsen, Mr David Bramley, and Mr Anthony Hazzard in the preparation of the book is gratefully acknowledged.

The present text is a draft for review and field-testing. The World Health Organization welcomes the comments of health professionals and other readers and users of this document.

WHO would like to acknowledge with thanks the financial support of the Opec Fund for International Development, Vienna, Austria, in the production of this book. This book has been developed in collaboration with the WHO Task Force for Cholera Control and the Swiss Disaster Relief Unit, Berne, Switzerland.

Introduction

Foodborne diseases, especially those caused by pathogenic organisms, remain a serious problem in all countries. Diarrhoea is a feature of most of these diseases and up to 70% of all episodes of diarrhoea may result from the ingestion of contaminated food and water.

The WHO book *Foodborne diseases: a focus for health education* underlines the importance of the education of consumers and food handlers, both domestic and professional, in food safety. It urges governments to take the initiative to develop, in collaboration with industries and consumers, a comprehensive, systematic and continuous programme of health education based on modern approaches to food safety. The book also identifies the health care system, particularly the primary health care system, as one of the most important vehicles for health education in food safety.

To be able to assume their role in food safety and advise the population on safe food preparation, health workers should know about the epidemiology of the principal foodborne diseases and the sociocultural conditions that encourage them. They should also receive some training in research methodology, especially in the investigation of foodborne disease outbreaks, Hazard Analysis and Critical Control Point (HACCP) studies, and the investigation of sociocultural characteristics of the population. Health workers should also be inspired to take action in their daily work to raise public awareness of food safety, to advise the mothers of small children or pregnant women in safe food preparation, and generally to assist the community in improving food safety.

To facilitate the training of health workers, WHO has developed a training package including this book and an accompanying training manual. The training package is intended for professionals in the

Introduction

health and environmental fields, particularly trainers of primary health care workers, physicians, nurses, midwives, nutritionists, medical students, and other professionals who need a basic understanding of food safety.

This book provides an introduction to the basic knowledge that health professionals need in order to discharge their responsibilities in food safety.

The book aims to increase the knowledge of health professionals regarding:

- the nature of foodborne diseases and their health and economic consequences;

- the epidemiology of foodborne diseases;

- the role of food in the transmission of various infections and intoxications;

- the factors leading to foodborne diseases;

- the measures necessary to improve food safety.

A training manual based upon a problem-solving approach to learning accompanies the present book. It provides direction on expected learning outcomes, summaries of key information to be covered, lists of recommended references and resources required, and suggestions for training activities. It also includes transparency masters and copies of hand-outs.

Chapter 1
Foodborne illness

Food in health and disease

Food is essential both for growth and for the maintenance of life. It supplies the energy and materials required to build and replace tissues, to carry out work and to maintain the body's defences against disease.

Food can also be responsible for ill-health. Failure to consume enough of the right kind of food will impede growth and impair health. For example, protein-energy malnutrition can lead to a range of clinical manifestations. These vary from marasmus, where consumption of protein, dietary energy and other nutrients are chronically reduced, to kwashiorkor (sometimes thought to be associated with an over-reliance on low protein staples) which results in a quantitative and qualitative deficiency of protein (Table 1.1).

Even when a diet provides enough protein and energy, it may not supply sufficient essential minerals or vitamins and may thus give rise to characteristic deficiency disorders (Table 1.2).

Illness can also result from what a food contains rather than from what it lacks. Some hazards of this kind are described as being intrinsic to the food in the sense that they are normal and natural constituents of the food. Many common food plants, for instance, contain toxic compounds designed to deter predators or invading microorganisms. Their intake is inevitably higher in those people with a largely vegetarian diet.

However, in most cases where the food supply is generally varied and plentiful,

Table 1.1 *Classification of severe protein-energy malnutrition in children*

Weight for age*	With oedema	Without oedema
60–80%	Kwashiorkor	Undernutrition
Less than 60%	Marasmic kashiorkor	Marasmus

* As % of standard (National Centre for Health Statistics) weight
Source: Tomkins, AM Nutrition in clinical medicine. In: Textbook of Medicine. RL Souhami and J Maxham (eds) 2nd edn. Churchill Livingstone, Edinburgh, 1994: p.106.

Table 1.2 *Examples of vitamin and mineral deficiency syndromes*

Micronutrient	Deficiency syndrome
A	Night blindness, xeropthalmia
Thiamine	Beriberi, Wernicke's encephalopathy; Korsakoff's psychosis
Niacin	Pellagra
Riboflavin	Mucosal lesions
Pyridoxine	Glossitis, neuropathy
Folate	Megaloblastosis, villus atrophy
B_{12}	Pernicious anaemia, megaloblastosis, neuropathy
C	Scurvy
D	Rickets, osteomalocia
K	Hypoprothrombinaemia
Iodine	Goitre, cretinism
Iron	Anaemia

and established processing and handling procedures are followed, the majority do not cause serious problems. Natural food toxins are described in more detail in Chapter 2 but a few examples are given in Table 1.3 and estimates for some mean daily intakes in the United Kingdom are presented in Table 1.4.

Other foodborne hazards can be described as extrinsic, indicating that their presence is a result of contamination of the food. This includes contamination with industrial chemicals or pesticide residues, right through to the presence of pathogenic bacteria or parasites. The range of possibilities is summarized in Table 1.3.

Table 1.3 *Causes of foodborne illness*

	Examples
INTRINSIC HAZARDS	
(Natural Toxins or Antinutritional Factors)	oxalic acid (rhubarb, spinach)
	alkaloids
	solanine (potatoes)
	dioscorine (yams)
	cyanide (cassava, lima beans)
	haemagglutinin (red kidney beans)
	protease inhibitors (legumes)
	phytic acid (bran)
	amatoxin, psilocybin and others
	(toxic mushroom)
EXTRINSIC HAZARDS	
Chemical Contamination	dioxins, PCBs
	heavy metals
	cadmium
	mercury
	lead
	pesticide residues
Biological Contamination	Bacteria
	causing infection e.g. *Salmonella*
	causing intoxication e.g. *C. botulinum*
	Parasites
	helminths e.g. roundworms
	protozoa e.g. *Giardia lamblia*
	Viruses e.g. Hepatitis A, Small Round-Structured Viruses (SRSVs)
	Fungi/mycotoxins e.g. aflatoxin
	Algae (e.g. dinoflagellates leading to paralytic shellfish poisoning)

Table 1.4 *Mean daily intakes (mg) of natural food toxicants*

Class of compound (food source)	Population	
	Total	Vegetarian
Glucosinolates (brassicas)	50	110
Glycoalkaloids (potatoes)	13	70 - 90
Saponins (legumes)	15	100 (*220)
Isoflavones (soya)	<1	105

* U.K. vegetarian population of East African origin
Source: Morgan, MRA. and Fenwick, GR National foodborne toxicants. Lancet, 15 December 1990, p. 1492/1495.

In most cases foods are not contaminated intentionally but rather from carelessness or insufficient education or training in food safety. In some cases, contamination may be deliberate as, for example, in the misuse of food additives such as prohibited colouring. In one serious case in Spain, contaminated industrial rapeseed oil was sold for human consumption, killing more than 500 people and crippling more than 20,000 (1).

How the relative importance of these hazards is perceived depends on who you ask. Surveys indicate that, as far as the general public is concerned, hazards associated with pesticide residues, environmental chemical contaminants and the use of food additives cause most concern. Yet experience shows that most outbreaks of foodborne disease are associated with microbiological contamination.

This is reflected in the available statistics on the etiology of foodborne illness. (Table 1.5). One study estimated that people are 100,000 times more likely to become ill as a result of microorganisms in food than as a result of pesticide residues (2).

Table 1.5 *Etiology of foodborne disease outbreaks (with known etiology) in Latin America and the Caribbean, 1995-1997*

Etiological agent	Percentage of outbreaks	Percentage of cases involved in outbreaks
Bacteria	46.3	83.03
Of which:		
Bacillus cereus	1.3	1.2
Clostridium perfringens	4.2	4.1
Clostridium botulinum	0.4	0.1
Escherichia coli	11.4	7.8
Salmonella	37.0	43.1
Shigella spp.	3.1	21.9
Staphylocccus aureus	36.6	19.5
Vibrio cholerae	4.2	0.9
Vibrio parahemolyticus	0.2	0.4
Other	1.6	1.0
Total	100.0	100.0
Viruses	1.8	3.7
Parasites	1.8	2.9
Marine toxins	44.2	8.0
Plant toxins	0.4	0.1
Chemical substances	5.4	2.3
Total	100.0	100.0

Source: Adapted from data provided by the Pan American Institute for Food Protection and Zoonoses, INPPAZ, PAHO/WHO 1998

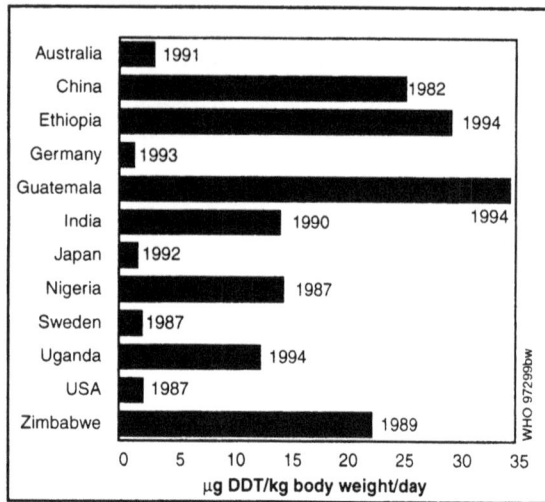

DDT complex (DDT and its degradation products) contaminates food mainly as a result of its earlier use in agriculture and public health. While DDT is now banned in most countries for agricultural uses, the persistence and fat solubility of DDT have resulted in widespread contamination of the food chain. Levels of DDT in breast milk reflect the exposure of the mother to DDT and is a good indicator of the levels of DDT in the food supply. Breast milk is also the sole food for the first few months of life and dietary intake of DDT complex by infants in some countries approaches or exceeds the WHO recommended provisional tolerable intake of 20 µg DDT/kg body weight/day.

Source: GEMS/Food WHO document (WHO/FSF/FOS/97.9)

Figure 1.1 *Dietary intake of DDT by infants from human milk*

Data collected by the Food Contamination Monitoring and Assessment Programme (GEMS/Food) indicate that in many countries the trend in chemical contaminant levels is generally downwards. This is most apparent in developed countries where exposure to these contaminants is often much lower than in developing countries (Figure 1.1).

Factors contributing to this disparity are discussed in Chapter 2. The general overall improvement is due to increased restriction of the use of toxic chemicals and pesticides that persist in the environment, and improved control of environmental pollution. Available data on foodborne illness of biological origin provide a strong contrast to this reduction in chemical contamination.

Several different types of organism can cause foodborne illness. Bacteria, single-celled organisms with typical dimensions of around $1\mu m$ ($10^{-6}m$), are the most important and well studied foodborne pathogens. A key factor is their ability to multiply in food, thus increasing the hazard they pose. This is discussed in Chapter 2. Filamentous fungi (moulds) can also grow in foods and some produce toxic substances called mycotoxins.

A number of human viruses can be transmitted by food and human diseases caused by protozoa, helminths and nematodes that are animal parasites are problems of emerging importance in a number of countries. These differ from most bacterial foodborne illnesses in that the causative organism does not multiply in the food itself. A brief description of the major foodborne pathogens and some of their key features is presented as Appendix 1. Most of the following is concerned primarily with bacterial pathogens, though specific aspects of other pathogens are mentioned where appropriate.

Extent of foodborne illness

Many developed countries have sophisticated systems for collecting data on the incidence and causes of foodborne illness. Yet it is known that these data represent only a fraction of the number of cases that occur. Infected individuals may not seek medical advice, and if they do their illness may not be recognized as foodborne in origin or may not be reported to the relevant authority for recording. Estimates vary but it is generally believed that in developed countries less than 10%, or even only 1%, of cases of foodborne illnesses ever reach official statistics. In countries with fewer resources, under-reporting must be even greater, with probably less than 1% of cases being reported. Studies in some countries point to an under-reporting factor of up to 350 in some cases.

Statistics from both developed and developing countries show an increasing trend in foodborne illness over recent years (Figure 1.2). In part, this is probably due to improvements in the way the

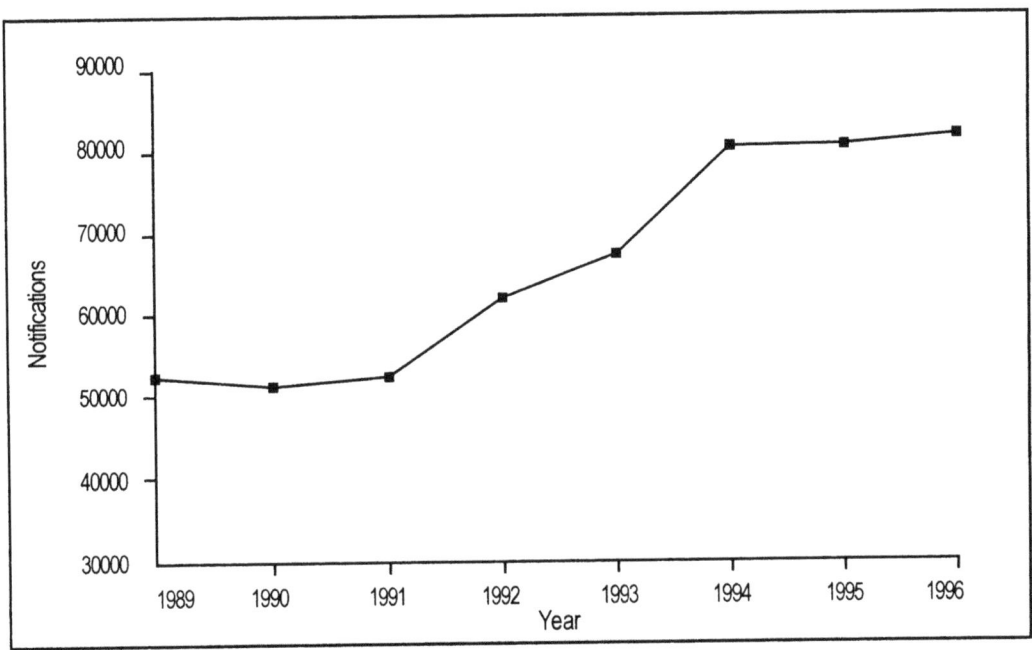

Figure 1.2a *Foodborne illness : annual notifications, England and Wales*

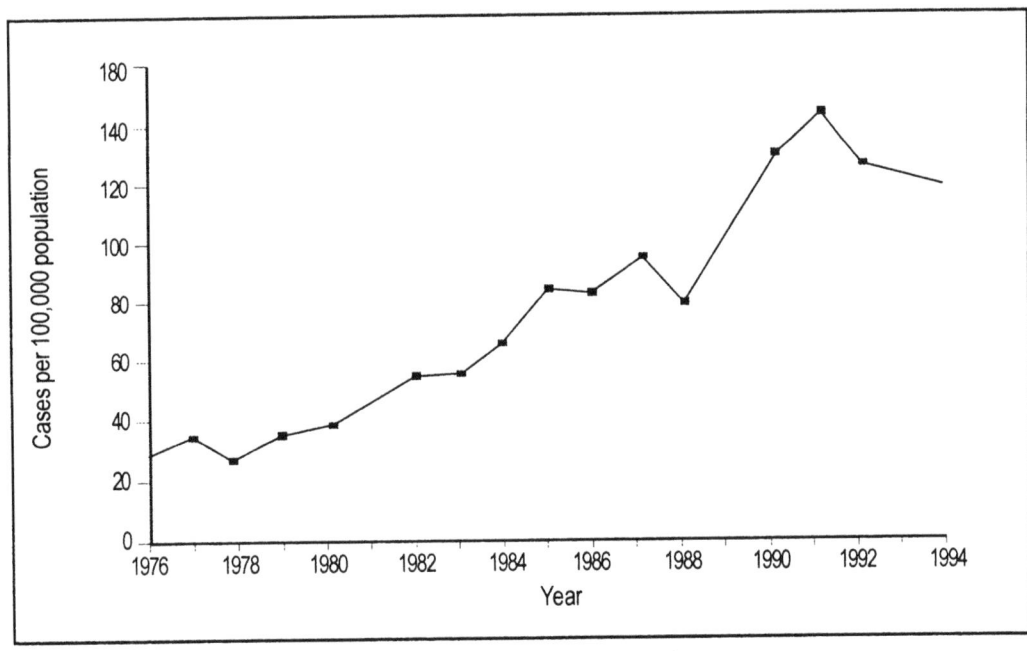

Figure 1.2b *Incidence of foodborne disease in Venezuela*

figures are collected, but it is thought to reflect an underlying increase in the number of cases as well.

A number of factors have contributed to this trend. Their relative importance varies between countries and between pathogens but some of the most significant are as follows:

- Increasing industrialization and urban living has meant that the food chain has become longer and more complex, increasing opportunities for contamination. It also means that more people are likely to be affected by a single breakdown in food hygiene.

- In poorer countries increased urbanization and rapid population growth have not been matched by development of the health-related infrastructure, including basic sanitation, and this has led to increased risk of contamination of the food and water supply.

- Increasing affluence in other areas has led to greater consumption of foods of animal origin such as meat, milk, poultry and eggs. These foods are recognized as more common vehicles of foodborne pathogens and this situation can be exacerbated by the methods of intensive production required to supply a larger market.

- There is greater international movement of both foods and people. Exotic *Salmonella* serotypes have been introduced into Europe and the United States as a result of the importation of animal feeds. A number of outbreaks of illness associated with imported foods have also been recorded. Tourism is one of the world's major growth industries and every year more and more people travel abroad where they are exposed to increased risk of contracting foodborne illness.

- Changing lifestyles also means that food preparation may be in the hands of the relatively inexperienced as more mothers go out to work and more people eat pre-prepared foods, meals from catering establishments or food from street vendors.

- An increasing proportion of the population is more susceptible to foodborne illness. This includes the malnourished, the elderly, those who have some underlying condition such as liver disease and those who are immunocompromised as a result of infections such as HIV and immunosuppressive medical treatment.

Foodborne illness: its definition and nature

The term "food poisoning" has often been used in some countries, but it is an expression that can sometimes be restrictive or misleading. *Foodborne illness* or *foodborne disease* are now the generally preferred terms. Foodborne disease can be defined as:

> "any disease of an infectious or toxic nature caused by or thought to be caused by the consumption of food or water".

Though there are a number of important exceptions that will be described later, in most cases and in most people's minds, the illnesses caused by foodborne microorganisms, principally bacteria, are associated with gastrointestinal symptoms of nausea, vomiting, stomach pains and diarrhoea. Since diarrhoea is a common clinical symptom in foodborne diseases, many of these diseases are referred to as "diarrhoeal diseases". These occur when the normal functions of the gut are upset in some way.

The gastrointestinal tract or gut is not an internal organ of the body but a tube running through it where foods are digested and absorbed, and unwanted waste products are expelled. In addition to absorption of nutrients from foods, absorption and secretion of water are important gut functions. Water absorption normally exceeds secretion. Each day, a typical adult will ingest about two litres of water. To this must be added saliva and secretions from the stomach, pancreas and liver which altogether make a total of 8-10 litres entering the small intestine daily. About 90% of this fluid is absorbed before it enters the large intestine where 80-90% of the remainder is absorbed. Changes in the small intestine that either decrease absorption or increase secretion will reduce overall absorption and result in a larger fluid flow into the large intestine. If this exceeds the relatively limited absorptive capacity of the large intestine then diarrhoea occurs.

Bacteria cause foodborne illness by two mechanisms: infection and intoxication. The latter can also be caused by chemical contaminants and naturally occurring toxins.

Infection

Infection occurs when living bacteria are ingested with food in numbers sufficient for some to survive the acidity of the stomach, one of the body's principal protective barriers. These survivors then pass into the small intestine where they multiply and produce symptoms.

Infections can be invasive or non-invasive. In non-invasive infections, the organism attaches itself to the gut surface or epithelium to prevent itself from being washed out by the rapid flow of material through the gut. It then multiplies, colonizing the surface. In some cases, such as infection with enteropathogenic *Escherichia coli*, this produces changes in the gut epithelium which reduce its absorptive capacity or cause fluid secretion. Colonizing bacteria can also produce enterotoxins; toxins that alter the function of the cells lining the gut and cause them to secrete water and electrolytes into the intestine to produce a profuse watery diarrhoea. A notable example of this is cholera, but a similar sequence of events occurs with enterotoxigenic *E. coli* infections.

Invasive pathogens are not confined to the intestinal lumen but can penetrate the cells lining the gut. In some cases their penetration is limited to the immediate vicinity of the gut, as with the non-typhoid salmonellas. Some pathogens invade the mucosa of the large intestine rather than the small intestine, producing inflammation, superficial abscesses and ulcers, and the passage of dysenteric stools containing blood, pus and large amounts of mucus. In other cases, microbial invasion is not restricted to the gut's immediate locality and the organism spreads further through the body, producing symptoms other than diarrhoea at sites remote from the gut itself, as for example in brucellosis, listeriosis, typhoid and paratyphoid fevers.

Illnesses caused by foodborne viruses and parasites are also broadly similar in that viable organisms gain access to their site of action in the body via the gastrointestinal tract.

Intoxication

With foodborne intoxications, the bacteria grow in the food producing a toxin. When the food is eaten, it is the toxin, rather than the microorganisms, that causes symptoms.

Since the toxin is ingested with the food there is no direct person-to-person spread, as can occur with some enteric infections, and the incubation period (the time between consumption of the food and the appearance of symptoms) tends to be shorter, generally of the order of one or two hours or even less in some cases. This is because the toxin begins to act as soon as it reaches the site of action, whereas with infections the microorganisms need time to multiply in the body.

There are some similarities here with other biotoxins such as mycotoxins and algal toxins, though algae differ from toxigenic bacteria and moulds in that they do not multiply in the food. Also, the health effects of mycotoxins tend to be long-term rather than acute (see Chapter 2).

Infectious dose

Infective pathogens can be introduced into the body from a variety of sources. In the past, it was thought that contaminated water was the main source of the pathogens that cause diarrhoea. This is probably still true in many cases, but it has been shown more recently that food may also be the vehicle of contamination in up to 70% of cases.

To cause illness, a sufficient number of cells must be consumed. This is known as the infectious dose. The infectious dose varies from one organism to another and from person to person. For *Campylobacter jejuni* the infectious dose is thought to be quite low, while relatively high numbers of non-typhoid *Salmonella* are normally required to produce illness. Experiments have been conducted where volunteers have consumed different levels of pathogens in order to determine the infectious dose. These results and data from the investigation of actual outbreaks give some indication of the numbers of bacteria required to produce illness, but they should be regarded only as a rough guide (Table 1.6).

Successful infection is the result of the interaction of two variable factors: the virulence of the pathogen (its ability to cause illness) and the susceptibility of the individual. The virulence of different *Salmonella* serotypes, for example, can

Table 1.6 *Estimated infectious doses*

Escherichia coli			
enteropathogenic	10^6–10^{10}		
enterotoxigenic	10^6–10^8		
enteroinvasive	10^8		
enterohaemorrhagic	10^1–10^3		
Shigella	10^1–10^2		
Salmonella Typhi	<10^3		
Other salmonellae	10^5–10^7		
but			
Salmonella Newport		60 – 230	in hamburger
Salmonella Eastbourne		10 – 25	in chocolate
Salmonella Heidelberg		100 – 500	in cheese
Clostridium perfringens	10^6–10^8		
Campylobacter	500		
Vibrio cholerae	10^6		
Vibrio parahaemolyticus	10^5–10^7		

differ appreciably. *Shigella* and enterotoxigenic *E. coli* (ETEC) are otherwise very similar organisms but estimates of their respective infective doses are markedly different, reflecting differences in their virulence.

Susceptibility to infection can vary with a range of factors such as age, general health, nutrition, immune status and whether a person is undergoing medical treatment. Listeriosis can be mild or even asymptomatic in some individuals but can be severe and often life-threatening in the unborn child. In people with low gastric acidity, increased survival of ingested pathogens can reduce the required infective dose, thereby increasing the risk of infection. This is often found in the elderly and may help explain their increased susceptibility to foodborne infections. The food that is the vehicle of infection may also help reduce the infectious dose by protecting the pathogen from the lethal effect of the stomach's acidity. This has been noted particularly with fatty foods such as salami, cheese, chocolate and ice cream where low numbers of salmonella have been implicated in foodborne disease outbreaks (Table 1.6).

Where the infectious dose is high, the food vehicle can play a very specific role in the illness. Depending on the food's composition and conditions of storage, a pathogen present at low and possibly harmless levels may grow to numbers sufficient to produce illness. The speed with which bacteria can grow is described in more detail in Chapter 2.

Health consequences of foodborne illness

For most adults in the industrialized world, incidents of foodborne illness are unpleasant but are generally mild and self-limiting indispositions that are restricted to gastroenteritis and are not usually life-threatening. Exceptions occur with particularly susceptible individuals such as the very old or very young, pregnant women or those who are already very sick or weak for some other reason. These vulnerable groups constitute quite a large proportion of the population and for many of them diarrhoeal disease can be fatal.

A number of foodborne pathogens such as *Clostridium botulinum* are also associated with acute extraintestinal (systemic) disease. *C. botulinum* causes a severe neuroparalytic syndrome which is often fatal. The mortality rate in outbreaks in the United States between 1976 and 1984 was 7.5% but it can be substantially higher (*3*). Survival in cases of botulism is critically dependent on early diagnosis and treatment.

Sometimes extra-intestinal disease transmitted by food is particularly associated with certain susceptible individuals. For example, infection by *Listeria monocytogenes* can vary from a mild, flu-like illness to meningitis and meningoencephalitis. It is particularly serious in pregnant women; the mother may experience relatively mild symptoms but infection of the fetus can result in abortion, stillbirth or premature labour. Listeriosis is also more than 300 times more common in AIDS patients than in the general population. Cancer patients and other immunocompromised individuals are subject to bacteraemia caused by foodborne bacteria. Verotoxin-producing *E. coli* generally results in a bloody diarrhoea but can cause the haemolytic uraemic syndrome, characterized by thrombocytopaenia, haemolytic anaemia and acute kidney failure, particularly in children.

Some chronic diseases, particularly arthritic conditions, can be triggered by

Table 1.7 *Examples of secondary disease state resulting from foodborne infections*

Disease	Associated complication
Brucellosis	Aortitis, orchitis, meningitis, pericarditis, spondylitis
Campylobacteriosis	Arthritis, carditis, cholecystitis, colitis, endocarditis, erythema nodosum, Guillain-Barré syndrome, haemolytic-uraemic syndrome, meningitis, pancreatitis, septicaemia
E.coli (EPEC & EHEC types) infections	Erythema nodosum, haemolytic-uraemic syndrome, seronegative arthropathy
Listeriosis	Meningitis, endocarditis, osteomyelitis, abortion and stillbirth, death
Salmonellosis	Aortitis, cholecystitis, colitis, endocarditis, orchitis, meningitis, myocarditis, osteomyelitis, pancreatitis, Reiter's syndrome, rheumatoid syndromes, septicaemia, splenic abscess, thyroiditis
Shigellosis	Erythema nodosum, haemolytic-uraemic syndrome, peripheral neuropathy, pneumonia, Reiter's syndrome, septicaemia, splenic abscess, synovitis
Taeniasis	Arthritis
Toxoplasmosis	Foetus malformation, congenital blindness
Yersiniosis	Arthritis, cholangitis, erythema nodosum, liver and splenic abcesses, lymphadenitis, pneumonia, pyomositis, Reiter's syndrome, septicaemia, spondylitis, Still's disease

Source: Mossel, 1988.

foodborne microorganisms (Table 1.7). In an outbreak of salmonellosis in Chicago in 1985, caused by contaminated pasteurized milk, more than 2% of the 170,000-200,000 people infected suffered from reactive arthritis as a result of their infection (*3*). Guillain-Barré syndrome is a serious and potentially life-threatening neurological disease characterized by acute weakness, autonomic dysfunction and respiratory insufficiency. It is a chronic sequela associated with acute gastrointestinal infection particularly by *Campylobacter jejuni*.

In developing countries, diarrhoeal diseases, particularly infant diarrhoea, are a major public health problem. It has been estimated that annually some 1500 million children under five years of age suffer from diarrhoea and over 3 million die as a result (*4*). Individual children experience on average 3.3 episodes of diarrhoea each year, though in some areas the number of episodes may exceed 9 and children can be suffering from diarrhoea for more than 15% of their young lives. The immediate cause of death from diarrhoeal disease is usually the dehydration that results from the loss of fluid and electrolytes in diarrhoeal stools, but diarrhoea can also have other serious health consequences. It may lead to malnutrition since food intake is reduced either as a result of loss of appetite or the withholding of food, and those nutrients that are ingested are poorly absorbed or simply lost by being swept out with the diarrhoeal stools. Malnutrition in its turn can predispose children to longer episodes of diarrhoea as well as other infections, aggravating the problem still further. This can result in a downward spiral of increasingly poor health which, unless it is broken in some way, will lead ultimately to premature death (Figure 1.3). Even where this does not proceed inexorably to a fatal end, the physical and mental growth of the child is severely impaired. This is shown in Figure 1.4 which records the effect of repeated bouts of diarrhoea and other illnesses on a child's development.

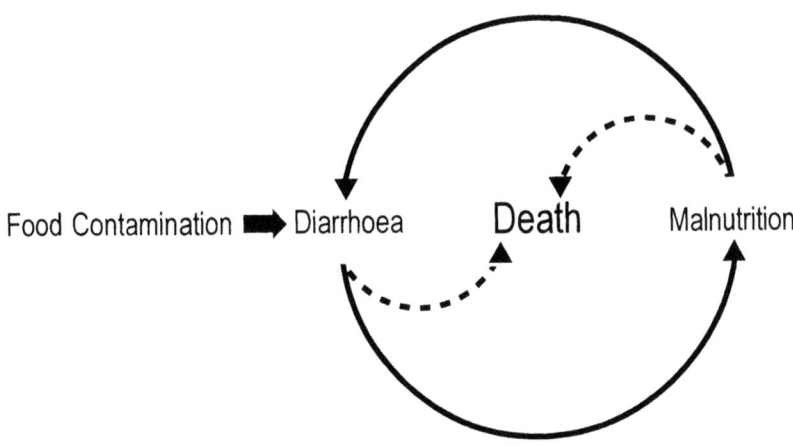

Figure 1.3 *The malnutrition and diarrhoea cycle*

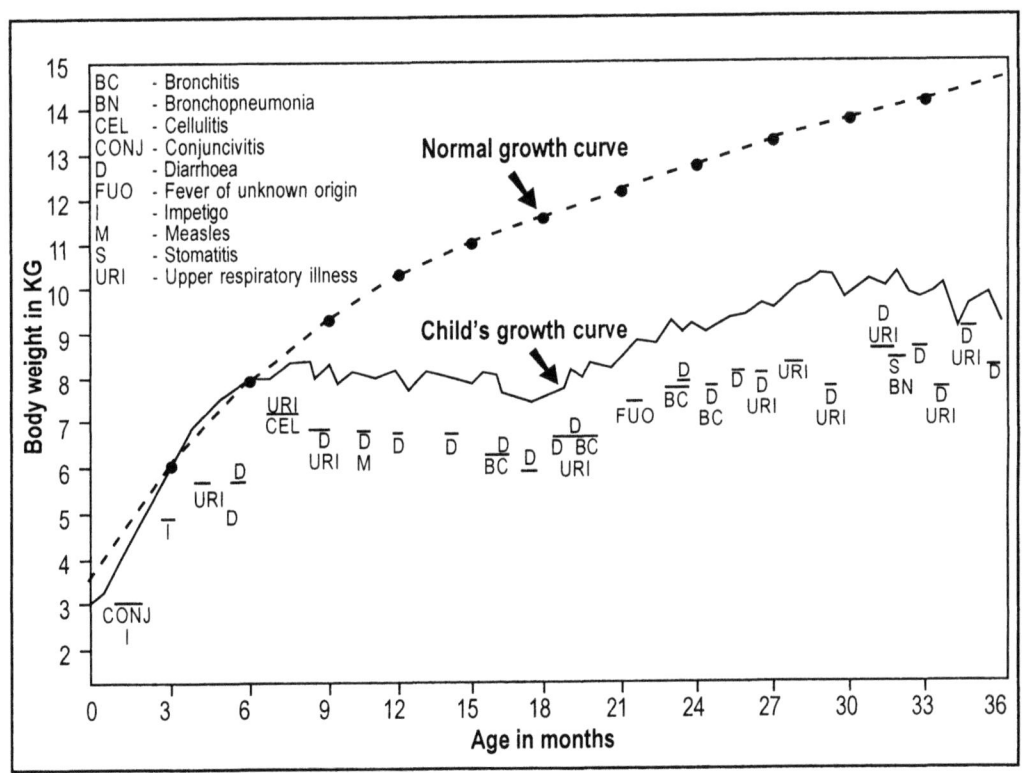

Source : Mata, LJ Nutrition and infection. Protein Advisory Group bulletin (1971)

Figure 1.4 *Growth pattern of a child with frequent episodes of diarrhoea and other infections* (The horizontal bars indicate the duration of the infectious disease)

Economic impact of foodborne illness

What is damaging and distressing at the level of the individual also has serious implications on a far larger scale. In developed countries efforts to quantify the economic impact of foodborne illness are comparatively recent, but it is clear from these that foodborne illness is a major burden on the economy. Costs arise from a number of different sources and are incurred both by the individual and by society at large. These costs include loss of income by the affected individual, cost of health care, loss of productivity due to absenteeism, costs of investigation of an outbreak, loss of income due to closure of businesses and loss of sales when consumers avoid particular products. In 1989 it was estimated that the total cost of bacterial foodborne illness to the United States economy was US$ 6,777,000,000. In developing countries, where the problem of diarrhoeal disease is far greater, the effect on economic activity and development can only be far more severe.

KEY POINTS

- Food is essential for health and well-being.

- Food may also be a cause of illness.

- Foods may be intrinsically toxic or may be contaminated with toxic chemicals or pathogenic organisms.

- Foodborne illness is extensively under-reported.

- Microorganisms (bacteria, viruses, moulds and parasites) are the most important cause of foodborne illness.

- Bacteria are generally most important.

- Most foodborne illness is associated with gastrointestinal symptoms of nausea, vomiting, stomach pains and diarrhoea.

- Foodborne illness is caused by two mechanisms: infection and intoxication.

- The infectious dose varies between organisms and between individuals.

- Foodborne illness can have seriously damaging effects on individuals, particularly young children, and on society as a whole.

Chapter 2
Foodborne hazards

Biological hazards

The overriding importance of microorganisms in foodborne illness has already been mentioned. Details of individual organisms are presented in Appendix 1. Here we briefly introduce the different types of organism responsible and then consider some general features associated with the transmission of microbial foodborne illnesses, particularly those caused by bacteria.

Parasites

These include protozoa and helminths (worms). Though considerably larger and more complex than other organisms conventionally classified as microorganisms, such as bacteria and viruses, it is often convenient to consider parasites under the same heading. Parasites can cause a variety of illnesses ranging from diarrhoea to liver cancer.

Infection with diarrhoeagenic protozoa such as *Giardia lamblia* and *Entamoeba histolytica* is normally the result of faecal contamination of a food or water source and direct person-to-person spread can occur. These protozoa can be killed by thorough cooking. Other protozoa such as *Toxoplasma gondii* and *Sarcocystis hominis* can infect the tissues of meat animals and be transmitted by undercooked meat.

Parasitic worms have complex life cycles where some time is spent in the tissues of an animal host (Figure 2.1). They do

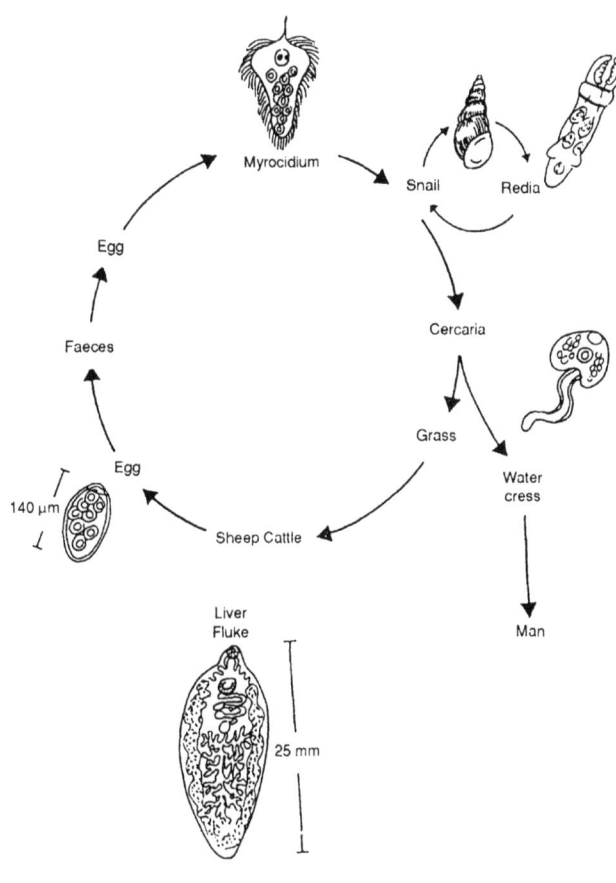

Figure 2.1 *Life cycle of the liver fluke, Fasciola hepatica*

not show any marked heat resistance and transmission to humans is usually the result of consumption of undercooked fish or meat. Some like the liver fluke *Fasciola hepatica*, however, spend part of their life cycle in a water snail from which it is released to contaminate aquatic plants which may then be eaten by humans. The pork and beef tapeworms *Taenia solium* and *T. saginata* respectively are widely distributed; in the Democratic Republic of Congo, Ethiopia and Kenya, more than 10% of the population are infected with *T. saginata*. In the former Yugoslavia up to 65% of children were found to harbour the organism (5). Foodborne trematode infections are a severe problem the extent of which is only just emerging (Figure 2.2).

Viruses

Viruses are very simple organisms that cannot replicate outside a susceptible host cell and do not therefore multiply in foods. Food and water can, however, be the vehicle for transmission of a number of different viruses that infect humans via the gastrointestinal tract. This is invariably the result of contamination of food by faeces or vomitus from an infected individual, possibly via some intermediary vehicle such as water or equipment.

Poliomyelitis and hepatitis A are the most serious viral diseases that are known to be transmitted by this route; Hepatitis E, which can be waterborne, is a significant cause of infectious hepatitis in Asia and Africa. There are also a number of food and waterborne viruses that cause diarrhoea, most notably the small round-structured viruses or Norwalk-like agents and Rotavirus.

Bacteria

Bacteria are generally considered to be the most important agents of foodborne illness. The individual organisms and the illnesses they cause are described in Appendix 1. Specific aspects of bacterial behaviour and foodborne illness feature prominently in Chapter 3.

Chemical hazards

For many chemical contaminants, a low level of consumption is both unavoidable and harmless. Various national regulatory authorities and international bodies, such as the Joint FAO/WHO Expert Committee on Food Additives (JECFA), have established threshold values for individual additives and contaminants below which there is no appreciable risk. These levels of acceptable daily intake (ADI) or provisional tolerable daily (or weekly) intake are expressed as the number of milligrammes of the chemical which may be safely consumed by a human for each kilogramme of the consumer's body weight. They are usually derived from experiments in animals which determine the level at which the chemical has no adverse effect on the animal. This is known as the no-observed-adverse-effect level (NOAEL). The NOAEL for the most sensitive animal species is then divided by a safety factor, usually 100, to arrive at the ADI. Bodies such as the Joint FAO/WHO Meeting on Pesticide Residues (JMPR) evaluate pesticide residues and recommend ADIs and maximum residue levels. Since its inception in 1962 the Joint FAO/WHO Codex Alimentarius Commission has adopted more than 3200 maximum residue levels for various pesticide/commodity combinations. Maximum residue levels are also prescribed for a number of veterinary drugs.

Chemical hazards in foods can arise from a number of different sources.

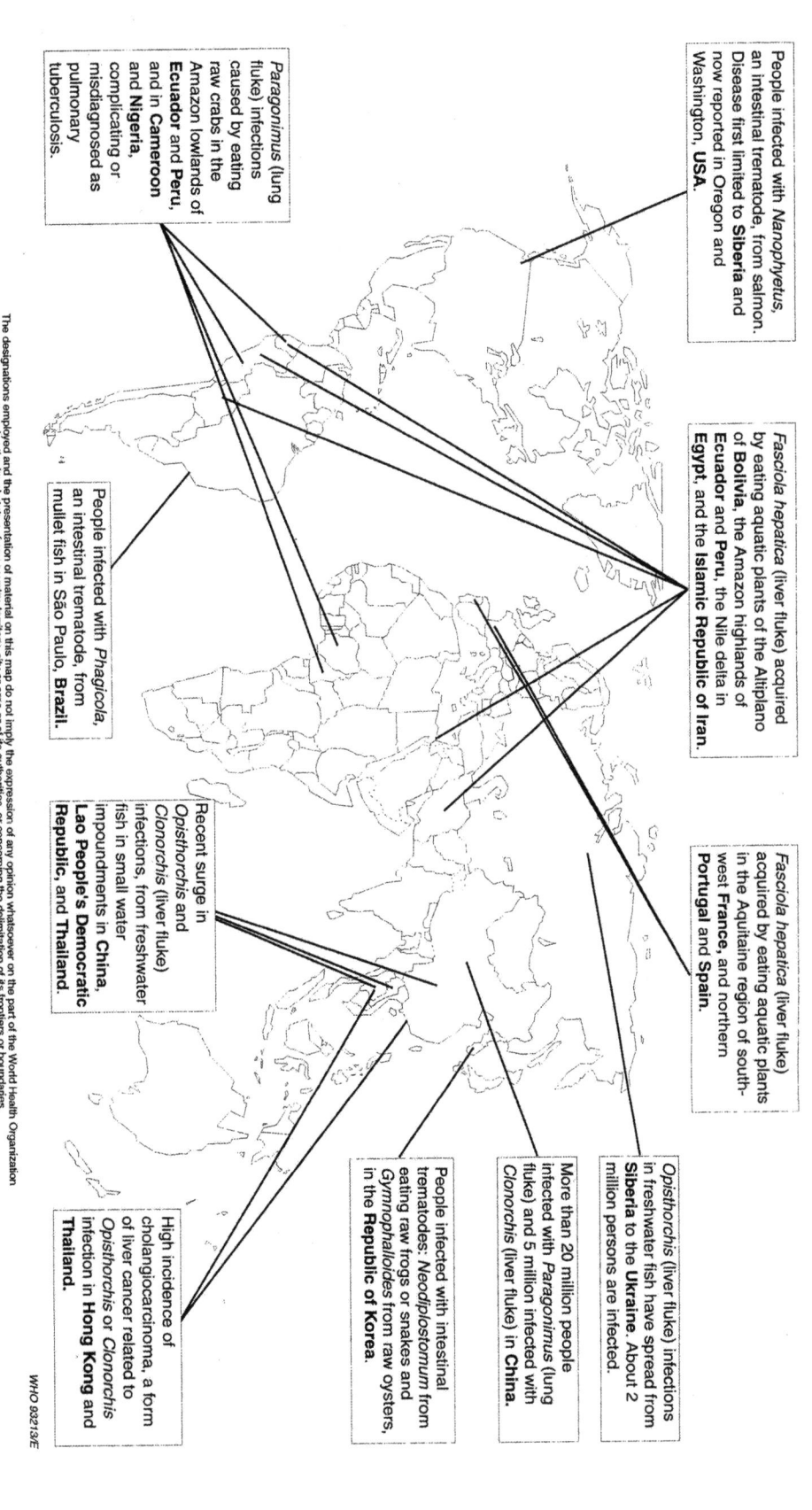

Figure 2.2 Foodborne trematode infections: the global distribution is changing with the environment and human behaviour

Industrial pollution of the environment

Modern industry produces huge numbers of chemical products and by-products. These can contaminate the environment and food chains, ultimately contaminating the human food supply itself. Most attention in this area has focused on heavy metals such as mercury, cadmium and lead, and organics such as polychlorinated biphenyls (PCBs). All are now widespread in the environment though their concentrations are usually low, except in cases of industrial accidents and environmental disasters.

Mercury, for example, has numerous industrial applications but also has toxic effects on animals and human beings, particularly pregnant women, nursing mothers and children. The most toxic form of mercury is methylmercury which damages the central nervous system. It is often found in fish since industrial effluents containing mercury are discharged into rivers or seas where the mercury is converted into methylmercury by bacteria. It then moves up the food chain and concentrates in the bodies of fish. The ability of contaminants or toxins to concentrate as they pass up the food chain is seen in numerous other instances. Pesticide accumulation is illustrated in Figure 2.3.

The most serious outbreak of mercury intoxication where industrial wastes contaminated fish occurred at Minimata Bay in Japan some years ago. Over 20,000 people are thought to have been poisoned since the outbreak was first recognized in 1956. Thirteen years later, fish in the bay still contained 50mg Hg/kg body weight compared with the Codex recommended limit of 0.5mg Hg/kg. In the Minimata case, contamination came from a single source but large quantities of mercury are also released from fossil fuel combustion, smelters and incinerators that can contaminate aquatic systems via the air. One example of this was when fish in lakes in northern Wisconsin in the USA were found to contain levels higher than 0.5mg/kg though they were remote from obvious sources of contamination.

Lead is a cumulative poison that affects the blood-forming tissues and the nervous and renal systems. Children are most susceptible and adverse effects on intelligence and behaviour have been seen with only very low levels of lead in the blood. Lead can be introduced into the environment by industry or in exhaust fumes from vehicles using leaded fuel. Sometimes the chemistry of the soil itself can give rise to contamination problems. A local cooking salt used by some villagers in Nigeria was found to contain very high levels of lead

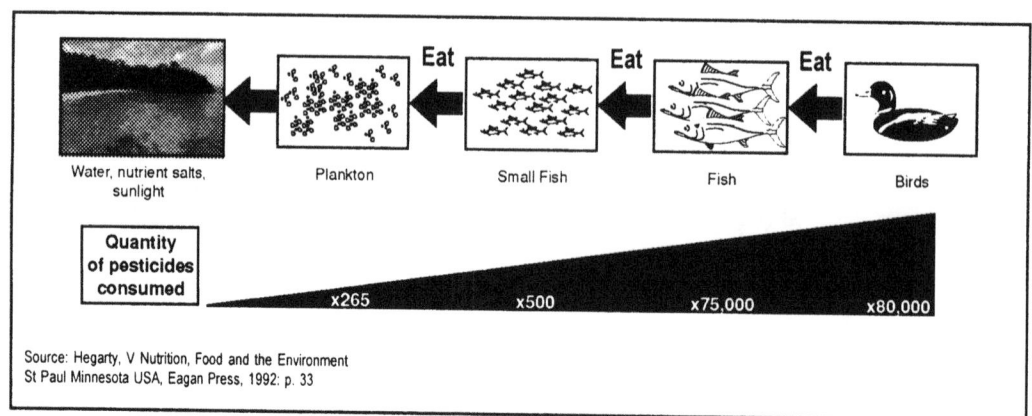

Source: Hegarty, V Nutrition, Food and the Environment
St Paul Minnesota USA, Eagan Press, 1992: p. 33

Figure 2.3 *Bioconcentration of environmental chemicals in the food chain*

(437 µg/kg) and manganese (2340 µg/kg) compared to common salt (1 µg lead/kg and 8.7 µg manganese/kg). Lead, silver and iron had been mined in the region and it was thought that the local geology led to high levels of these elements in the natural spring from which the salt was recovered (6).

PCBs were manufactured for industrial applications such as use in hydraulic systems, transformers and heat exchangers though their production has been drastically reduced in many countries since the 1970s. Contamination of edible oil with PCB has caused large-scale poisonings in Japan and Taiwan and exposure to PCB in the workplace has been associated with an increased risk of cancer. Exposure of women to PCBs during pregnancy appears to have a long-term impact on the intellectual function of their children (7). Fish generally contain higher levels of PCBs than other types of food. Information on dietary exposure to PCBs is almost exclusively from industrialized countries but the basic trend has been downwards since the 1970s.

Agricultural practices

Foods can also carry residues of pesticides and veterinary drugs. Organochlorine pesticides such as DDT, aldrin and dieldrin were identified in the early 1970s as a particular problem since they persist in the environment, accumulate in the fatty tissues and increase in concentration as they pass up the food chain (Figure 2.3). Contamination is particularly associated with foods such as milk, animal fats, fish and eggs. As a result of concerns over their potential carcinogenicity and harm to the environment, the use of organochlorine pesticides has been restricted in many countries and residue levels in foods have shown a decline over recent years. They do however remain important in many developing countries, where DDT for instance is still widely used in the fight against malaria. Residue levels in foods from developing countries are generally higher, but data are not available from many countries.

Organochlorine pesticides have increasingly been replaced by organophosphorus compounds. These do not persist in the environment or animal tissues for long periods and survey data have shown that they are seldom present in foods. However, they pose a serious health risk when ingested at high concentrations.

In a study of 63 outbreaks of intoxication due to pesticides (8) four causes of food contamination were identified:

■ *Contamination during transport or storage*

Typical cases involved powders such as sugar or flour which were transported or stored with a pesticide or in a place previously contaminated with pesticide.

■ *Ingestion of seed dressed for sowing*

Mainly associated with organic mercury fungicides, such outbreaks occurred particularly during times of food shortage when treated seeds were distributed after farmers had already sown their own grain. Local people were unable to read the warning label on the bags or mistakenly believed that washing off the dye also removed the pesticide.

■ *Mistaken use in food preparation*

This occurs when pesticides are mistaken for food materials such as sugar, salt and flour.

■ *Misuse in agriculture*

Pesticides have been found in food or water due to misuse near harvesting time, misuse of containers, contamination of ground water and use of excessively high doses in agriculture.

Residues of veterinary drugs such as antibiotics can also find their way into milk or meat. In many cases the long-term effects of these on human health are not known but they can, for example, provoke strong allergic reactions in sensitive people. They can also encourage the spread of antibiotic resistance in bacteria, making treatment of human infection more difficult, and for this reason it has been recommended that antibiotics used in human medicine should not be used in animals. Antibiotic residues in milk that is used to produce fermented products can interfere with the fermentation process by inhibiting the desirable lactic acid bacteria. Normally this is just a technical problem resulting in economic loss but, when it occurs, pathogens present in the milk may grow and pose a health hazard later. For these reasons many countries have regulations prohibiting the sale of milk from cows being treated for mastitis and milk is routinely tested for the presence of antibiotic residues.

A few hormonal agents are used for growth promotion in farm animals (e.g. bovine somatotropin hormone, or BST). Minute residues of these drugs do not pose a risk for consumers, although there are different opinions on the acceptability of these drugs and monitoring is necessary to ensure that permitted limits are not exceeded.

Food processing

Chemical contaminants can sometimes be introduced as a result of food processing and storage. Drinking water can be contaminated from lead used in water storage tanks and piping and this has on occasion caused cases of lead poisoning in children (9). Lead-based solder used in certain types of can is the major source of lead in canned foods, and processors in many countries have now adopted non-soldered cans as a simple remedy for this problem. Lead can also leach into foods stored in inadequately glazed earthenware pots. When pots are glazed at temperatures below 1200°C, much of the lead in the glaze will remain soluble and if the pots are used to store acidic foods such as pickles or fruit juices then the product can become contaminated. Apple juice that caused a fatal case of lead poisoning contained 1300 mg/l lead after three days storage in such a jar (10).

Chemicals have been deliberately added to foods since the earliest times. Before the advent of accurate analytical methods this was largely uncontrolled and open to abuse, but nowadays their use is subject to much closer regulation. Food additives can serve a number of purposes, such as preservative, antioxidant, acidity regulator, emulsifier, colour, flavour or processing aid. The health implications of additives is constantly under review by national regulators and international bodies such as JECFA who recommend ADI levels on the basis of data from toxicological studies. Additives such as some food colourings have occasionally been banned as a result of such studies. Where additives are allowed, permitted levels of use are prescribed for specified foods. Occasional problems may arise, however, with unscrupulous or ill-informed food processors who use non-permitted additives such as boric acid or excessive levels of permitted ones.

Nitrates and nitrites occur naturally in the environment and are also deliberately added to some processed foods as a preservative and colour fixative. They are, for example, particularly important for controlling the growth of *Clostridium botulinum* in cured meats. Under suitable conditions, the presence of nitrate/nitrite can lead to the formation of nitrosamines which are known to cause cancer in mammals. Studies have shown that food preparation techniques such as malting grain, smoking, drying and broiling of meat and fish and the frying of cured meats can, under certain conditions, promote the formation of nitrosamines.

To reduce exposure to these compounds, good manufacturing practices are recommended which include addition to foods of the minimum amounts of nitrates/nitrites necessary to achieve their functional purpose and the use of nitrosation inhibitors such as ascorbate.

Natural toxicants in foods

Many plants that serve as staple human foods often contain a range of secondary compounds that are produced to deter predators (Table 1.3). Over the years, selective plant breeding has to some extent reduced the level of these protective factors, though this of course increases the plant's vulnerability to pests and disease. Human ingenuity has also developed processing procedures that eliminate or at least reduce the hazard. Cooking of legumes, for example, can be important in destroying protease inhibitors and haemagglutinins (lectins) which, if ingested, can inhibit growth and sometimes cause illness.

Failure to recognize the significance of certain traditional food processing procedures can also lead to food safety problems. One good example of this is cassava which serves as the major source of dietary energy for about 500 million people worldwide. All cassava cultivars contain the cyanogenic glucosides, linamarin and lotaustralin. When the plant tissues are damaged, these compounds are attacked by the enzyme linamarase which degrades them to cyanohydrins which then decompose to release hydrogen cyanide. Processing of cassava which involves extended crushing and soaking of the roots maximizes conversion of the bound cyanide to its free form which is much easier to remove.

Konzo is a tropical myelopathy, characterized by the onset of spastic paraparesis, which occurs as epidemics in rural areas of Africa as a result of consuming insufficiently processed cassava. It can arise when rapidly growing populations experience declining agricultural yields and resort to cultivating high-yielding bitter cassava with high cyanogen levels, though other factors have also been shown to contribute. For example, in the Bandundu region of the Democratic Republic of Congo, construction of a new road improved transport to the capital and made cassava an important cash crop. To meet the higher demand, the women who were processing cassava reduced the soaking time from three days to one, resulting in higher cyanogen levels in the product. This led to outbreaks of konzo in the dry season when the diet tends to lack supplementary foods containing sulfur-amino acids which are essential for cyanide detoxification. Villages where the traditional three days soaking was retained did not report any konzo cases (11).

Glucosinolates are sulfur-containing compounds produced from amino acids. They occur particularly in cruciferous plants such as mustard, cabbage, broccoli, turnip and water cress where they contribute a pungency to the product's flavour. Cooking can reduce levels by up to 60%. In some cases, glucosinolates have been associated with hypothyroidism, endemic goitre, but problems with their toxicity appear to have been mostly associated with the growth impairment of farm animals. In contrast, a number of epidemiological studies have indicated that consumption of cruciferous vegetables is associated with a lower risk of tumour formation in the human digestive tract, suggesting that they exert a protective effect against carcinogenesis (12).

Favism is an acute haemolytic reaction found primarily around the Mediterranean

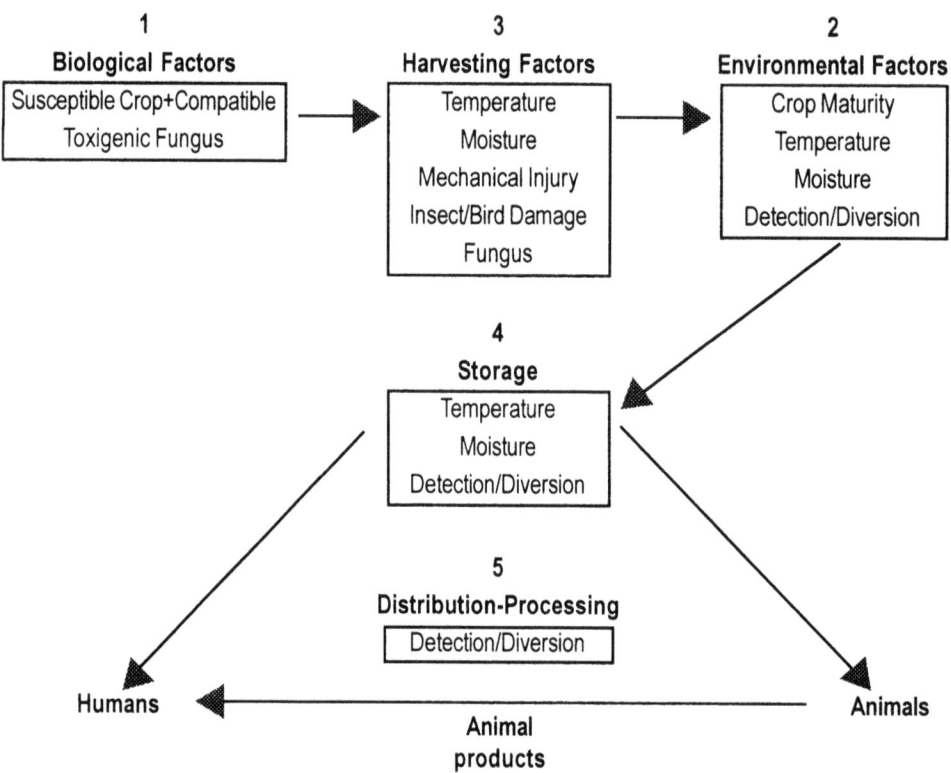

Figure 2.4 *Factors influencing the production of mycotoxins in foods*

and in the Middle East in people with an inherited deficiency of the enzyme glucose-6-phosphate dehydrogenase. It is triggered by exposure to fava beans (*Vicia fava*) and is thought to be caused by alkaloids such as vicine which occur in the skin of the bean.

Lathyrism, a condition characterized by a spastic paralysis of the legs, is associated with consumption of the pulse *Lathyrus sativus* in North Africa and Asia. It is caused by a neurotoxin which can be removed from the pulse by prolonged boiling in water. Its toxicity is well known but the plant is hardy and survives adverse conditions well. Outbreaks of illness are particularly associated with times of severe food scarcity when it can form a major part of the diet.

Solanine is a glycoalkaloid found in potatoes. Concentrations are highest in the sprouts and skin (especially when green) and it is not destroyed by cooking. It is an inhibitor of the enzyme cholinesterase and has been implicated in cases of human illness where the symptoms involve gastrointestinal upset and neurological disorders.

Biological sources

Mycotoxins

Some moulds have the ability to produce toxic metabolites, known as mycotoxins, which can produce a range of disorders from gastroenteritis to cancer. More than 300 mycotoxins have been identified but only a relatively small number have been shown to occur in foods and feeds at levels sufficient to cause concern. A list of these and some of their characteristics is presented as Table 2.1.

The aflatoxins are probably the most extensively studied mycotoxins. They were discovered in the United Kingdom in the early 1960s following the death of thousands of turkey poults which had con-

Table 2.1 *Toxicity and biological effects of some major mycotoxins found in foods*

Mycotoxin	Major Foods	Common producing spp.	Biological activity	LD$_{50}$ (mg kg^{-1})
Aflatoxins	Maize, groundnuts, figs, tree nuts (Aflatoxin M$_1$ (secreted by cow after metabolism of Afl B$_1$) Milk, milk products)	Aspergillus flavus Aspergillus parasiticus	Hepatotoxic, carcinogenic	0.5 (dog), 9.0 (mouse)
Cyclopiazonic acid	Cheese, maize, groundnuts, Rodo millet	Aspergillus flavus Penicillium aurantiogriseum	Convulsions	36 (rat)
Deoxynivalenol	Cereals	Fusarium graminearum Fusarium culmorum	Vomiting, feed refusal	70 (mouse)
T-2 toxin	Cereals	Fusarium sporotrichioides	Alimentary toxic aleukia	4 (rat)
Ergotamine	Rye	Claviceps purpurea	Neurotoxin	
Fumonisin	Maize	Fusarium moniliforme	Equine encephalomalacia pulmonary oedema in pigs oesophageal carcinoma	?
Ochratoxin	Maize, cereals, coffee beans	Penicillium verrucosum Aspergillus ochraceus	Nephrotoxic	20–30 (rat)
Patulin	Apple juice, damaged pomme fruits	Penicillium expansum	Oedema, haemorrhage possibly carcinogenic	35 (mouse)
Penitrem A	Walnuts	Penicillium aurantiogriseum	Tremorgen	1.05 (mouse)
Sterigmatocystin	Cereals, coffee beans, cheese	Aspergillus versicolor	Hepatotoxic, carcinogenic	166 (rat)
Tenuazonic acid	Tomato paste	Alternaria tenuis	Convulsions, haemorrhage	81 (female mouse) 186 (male mouse)
Zearalenone	Maize, barley, wheat	Fusarium graminearum	Oestrogenic	not acutely toxic

sumed feed containing groundnut meal contaminated by the mould *Aspergillus flavus*. Since the fungi producing aflatoxins are prevalent in areas of high humidity and temperature, crops in tropical and subtropical regions are more subject to contamination.

Aflatoxins are acutely toxic and have been shown to be carcinogenic for some animals. Their toxicity varies between different species but data from a large outbreak of poisoning in India in 1974, which involved mouldy maize and in which nearly 100 people died, suggests that the toxicity of aflatoxin B$_1$ for humans lies somewhere between that for the dog and that for the rat. The involvement of aflatoxins with human cancer is more complex and remains to be defined. For example, the risk of liver cancer is believed to increase with the prevalence of hepatitis B in the population (*13*).

The FAO has estimated that up to 25% of the world's foods are significantly contaminated with mycotoxins (*14*). They are produced by moulds infecting agricultural crops, particularly cereals and oilseeds, during both growth and post-harvest storage and their occurrence is the result of complex interactions between the toxinogenic organism, the host plant and a range of environmental factors (Figure 2.4). Mycotoxins can also occur in milk, meat and their products as a result of animals consuming mycotoxin-contaminated feed. Aflatoxin M$_1$ is a metabolite of aflatoxin B$_1$ which is itself thought to be carcinogenic and can be isolated from a cow's milk 12 hours after consumption of the aflatoxin B_1. It is unaffected by pasteurization treatments and will persist into products such as yoghurt, cheese and cream. It can also be isolated from human breast milk. However, it is thought to be considerably less potent than aflatoxin B_1.

Mycotoxins differ in their chemical and physical properties but most can be considered relatively stable to heat and other processes normally applied in the production and preparation of food. A number of countries have established limits for mycotoxins in particularly susceptible foods (Table 2.2).

Algal toxins

A number of algae can produce heat-resistant toxins which are not destroyed when the alga is eaten by a predator. The toxin can then be passed up the food chain and accumulated by other organisms which are eaten by people. Ciguatera poisoning, a sometimes fatal condition characterized by nausea, vomiting, diarrhoea and sometimes neurosensory disturbances, convulsions and paralysis, is the most common example with thousands of cases occurring each year in tropical and subtropical regions. Details of the etiology of ciguetera poisoning are described in Chapter 3.

Transmission of algal toxins to humans is often associated with the consumption

Table 2.2a *The range of regulatory limits for mycotoxins*

Mycotoxin	Reg. Limit (µg kg^{-1})	Number of Countries
Aflatoxins in foods	0*	48
Aflatoxin M_1 in milk	0*–1	17
Deoxynivalenol in wheat	1000–4000	5
Ochratoxin A in foods	1–300	6
Patulin in apple juice	20–50	10
T-2 Toxin	100	2
Zearalenone	30–1000	4

* Limit of determination

Table 2.2b *Maximum acceptable levels for aflatoxin for a selection of countries (Aflatoxin B, unless otherwise stated)*

Country	Limit (µg kg^{-1})	Foods
United Kingdom	2	Nuts, dried figs and their products
	5	As above but intended for further processing
United States	20	Total aflatoxins in all foods
	0.5	Aflatoxins M_1 in whole milk, low fat milk and skim milk
Australia	5	All foods except peanut products
	15	Peanut products
India	30	All foods
Japan	10	All foods
China	50	Rice, peanuts, maize, sorghum, beans, wheat, barley, oats

Table 2.3 *Principal algal intoxications associated with shellfish*

Syndrome	Symptoms	Toxin	Algal species
Amnesic shellfish poisoning	choking, vomiting, diarrhoea, incapacitating headaches, seizure and short-term memory loss	domoic acid	*Pseudonitzschia pungens*
Diarrhetic shellfish poisoning	diarrhoea, vomiting, abdominal pain, nausea (may persist for several days)	okadaic acid dinophysistoxin	*Dynophysis acuta* *Dynophysis acuminata* *Dynophysis fortii*
Neurotoxic shellfish poisoning	paresthesia, reversal of hot and cold temperature sensitivity myalgia and vertigo (generally mild)	brevetoxins	*Ptychodiscus brevis* (*Gymnodium breve*)
Paralytic shellfish poisoning	tingling, numbness in fingertips and lips, giddiness, staggering, incoherent speech, respiratory paralysis (high mortality rate)	saxitoxin gonyautoxin	*Alexandrium (Gonyaulax) catenella* *Alexandrium tamarensis*

of shellfish. More widespread than ciguatera intoxication, cases have been reported from locations all over the world. Four distinct syndromes are recognized and some of their features are described in Table 2.3.

For sufficient toxin to accumulate it is usually necessary for there to be a sudden increase or bloom of toxigenic algal species in a locality. This is usually a result of a combination of climatic conditions, light, salinity and nutrient supply and when it occurs the only preventive measure is to ban the harvesting and consumption of shellfish from these areas.

Physical hazards

At almost any stage in its production, food can be contaminated with foreign material that could be a physical hazard to the consumer. Physical hazards are very diverse and difficult to categorize since it is possible to conceive circumstances in which almost any foreign object could cause harm. Some, such as pieces of glass, pose an obvious risk of cutting the consumer's mouth or doing even greater damage if swallowed. For this reason, food manufacturers take great care to reduce the risk of this happening by restricting the use of glass in equipment and sheathing light fittings to prevent glass dropping into food in the event of a bulb or tube breaking. Often, of course, glass is the packing material of choice for foods and great care must be taken to avoid breakage or damage to containers that could result in slivers of glass being packed with the food. Sharp stones, pieces of metal, bone or wood can cause similar problems.

Any hard object can damage teeth and an even wider range of other, often apparently innocuous, objects can cause choking when swallowed. These often pose a particular risk for young children. To minimize such risks, commercial food manufacturers go to great lengths, installing devices such as metal detectors and X-ray machines to detect foreign objects in food, and controlling the quality of their raw materials and the production environment. Such measures are inappropriate to domestic food preparation where care and vigilance are the best ways to avoid physical hazards.

KEY POINTS

- Foodborne hazards can be classified as biological, chemical or physical.

- Biological hazards can be posed by parasites, viruses or bacteria.

- Chemical contaminants in foods can come from industrial and agricultural sources, from food processing or from the food itself.

- Toxic chemicals also come from biological sources such as moulds and algae.

- Foreign objects present in food could constitute a physical hazard to the consumer.

Chapter 3
Factors leading to microbial foodborne illness

Three key factors generally contribute to outbreaks of microbial foodborne illness:

- **contamination** - pathogens must be present in the food;
- **growth** - in some cases they must also have the opportunity to multiply in the food in order to produce an infectious dose or sufficient toxin to cause illness;
- **survival** - when present at a dangerous level they must be able to survive in the food during its storage and processing.

Contamination: how do microorganisms get into food?

Microorganisms, particularly bacteria, can be found almost everywhere. They are present in the air, water and soil; they can grow wherever higher organisms can grow, and can be found on the surfaces of plants and animals as well as in the mouth, nose and intestines of animals, including humans. They also occur in places that are far too inhospitable for higher life forms, such as in hot sulfur springs. As a result, foods are hardly ever sterile, that is to say completely free from viable microorganisms. Foods carry a mixed population of microorganisms derived from the natural microflora of the original plant or animal, those picked up from its environment and those introduced during harvest/slaughter and subsequent handling, processing and storage.

Most of the microorganisms in our environment cause us no harm. In fact they play very useful roles in making soil fertile and decomposing and recycling organic and inorganic materials that would otherwise accumulate. When they occur in foods, many of these organisms have no evident effect on the food or the person consuming it. In some cases, microorganisms may actually produce beneficial changes in the food and this is the basis of the large range of fermented foods such as cheese, yoghurt and fermented meats. Others, however, will spoil the product making it unfit for consumption and some can be harmful to humans causing illness when they or the toxins they produce are ingested.

Factors leading to microbial foodborne illness

It is possible to control and minimize the numbers of organisms present in food by using good hygienic practices in its preparation and handling or by processing the food in some way. If pathogens all came from the same source then the task of controlling them would be much simpler. Unfortunately they can get into foods from several different sources (Figure 3.1), known as reservoirs of infection, and by a number of routes.

Microorganisms that occur naturally in foods (indigenous microflora)

Food materials, plant and animal, will carry their own microflora during life and this can persist into the food product. In terms of food safety, the natural microflora is of greatest importance in animal products. The muscle of healthy animals and poultry is usually almost completely free from microorganisms but the intestines in particular carry a very large and diverse microflora that can include human pathogens such as *Campylobacter*, *Salmonella* and certain strains of *Escherichia coli*. In the process of slaughter and butchering a carcass, these organisms may be spread to other meat surfaces. As a result, evisceration and dressing are regarded as key steps that need to be hygienically performed to minimize meat contamination.

In most cases the animal or bird will carry these organisms without showing signs of ill-health, and pathological lesions will not be visible during meat inspection. Others, such as *Bacillus anthracis*, the causative agent of anthrax, can cause an illness in the animal and visible lesions. Since this and other animal diseases can be transmitted to humans, it is clear that meat from obviously sick animals must not be used as human food. Other diseases, such as bovine tuberculosis, brucellosis or the presence of parasites such as the beef and pork tapeworms and the roundworm *Trichinella spiralis*, may also be diagnosed during post mortem meat inspection. Thus ante and post mortem examination by a trained inspector is an essential protection measure.

Natural inhabitants of the environment

Many pathogens can be found as natural inhabitants of the environment — the soil, air and water where the food is produced — and can, as a result, contaminate the product. For example, *Vibrio parahaemolyticus* is a naturally occurring marine organism in warm coastal waters and can contaminate fish. Some strains are pathogenic and this can be a very important cause of foodborne illness where fish is a major item in the diet. *Clostridium botulinum* and *Clostridium perfringens* are

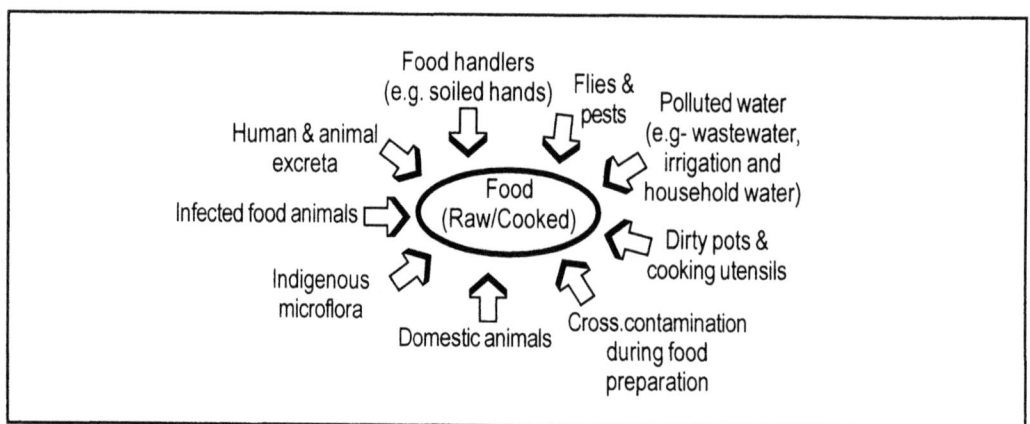

Figure 3.1 *Sources of food contamination*

found in soil and mud. *Bacillus cereus* spores can be isolated from soil and air, and *Listeria monocytogenes* is a relatively common environmental organism found in unpolluted water, mud and numerous other sources.

Polluted environment: insanitary practices in agriculture and aquaculture

Pollution of the environment with animal or human wastes such as sewage can be a serious threat to food safety. Human excrement can contain a wide range of pathogens transmitted by the faecal-oral route including bacteria such as *Vibrio cholerae*, *Salmonella* Typhi, viruses such as Hepatitis A, and parasites. These can be transferred to foods if raw sewage is used to fertilize fields or if the water used to irrigate, wash, cool or transport food is contaminated with sewage.

Filter-feeding shellfish will filter large volumes of water to extract nutrients. If this water is polluted with sewage they will also concentrate pathogenic bacteria and viruses in their tissues. Polluted water used in aquaculture can also lead to the carriage of pathogens such as *Vibrio cholerae* by farmed fish and shellfish.

Animal excrement poses equally serious problems. For example, a large outbreak of listeriosis was caused by the contamination of cabbages with sheep manure. Chicken faeces adhering to the outside of egg shells can contaminate the contents when the egg is broken and this has been the cause of numerous outbreaks of salmonellosis. Sometimes the link between the food and faecal contamination can be quite complex, as was illustrated by an outbreak of yersiniosis (Figure 3.2). In this case, crates used to transport waste milk to a farm where it was used as animal feed were contaminated with pig excrement. Back at the dairy, the

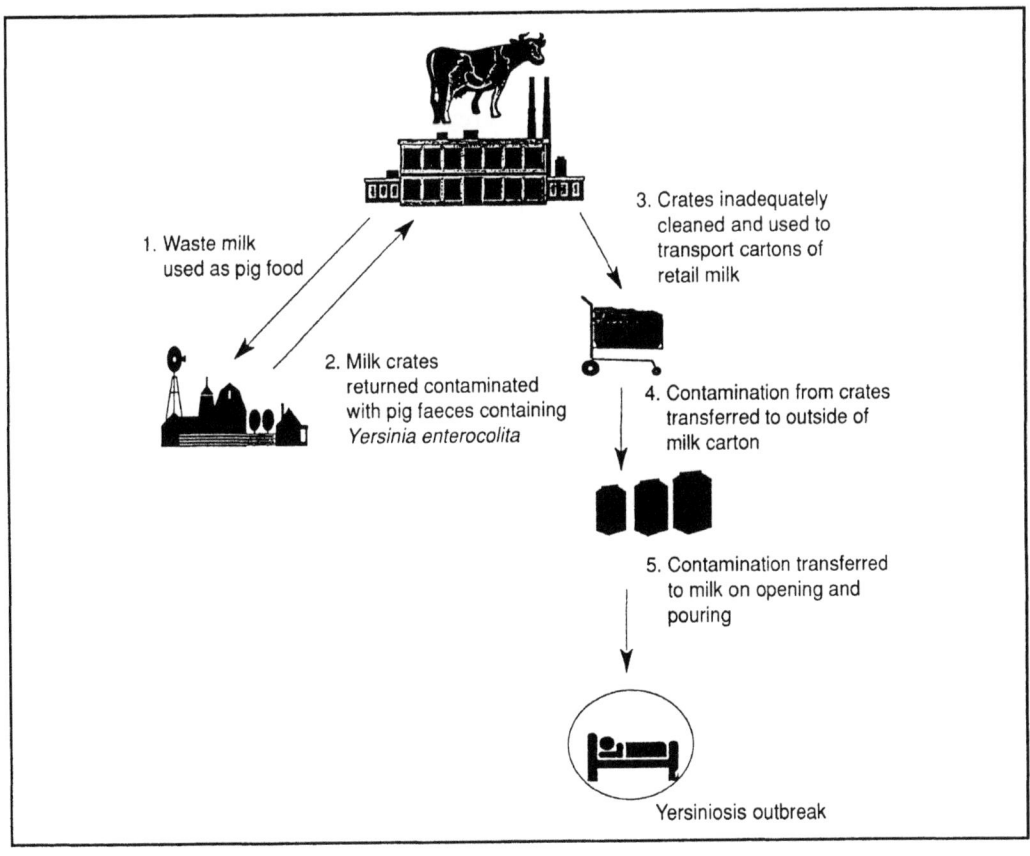

Figure 3.2 *Faecal contamination leading to an outbreak of yersiniosis*

crates were insufficiently washed and disinfected before being used to transport retail milk to the shops. During this process the outside of the milk cartons were contaminated with *Yersinia enterocolitica* which was, in turn, transferred to the milk when the cartons were opened and the milk poured.

Water

Contaminated water is simply one aspect of a polluted environment, but in view of its importance in foods and food processing and its role as a major source of diarrhoeal disease in developing countries it merits special mention. Contamination of water with faeces can introduce a wide variety of pathogenic bacteria, viruses, protozoa and helminths which can be transmitted to people when the water is used for drinking or in food preparation. Since individual water sources tend to serve large numbers of people, disease outbreaks where water is the primary source of infection can be very large. This linkage between water and the spread of disease has been known for a long time and is reputed to have been dramatically demonstrated in 1854 by John Snow when he removed the handle from a water pump in Broad Street, London, to bring a local cholera outbreak to an end.

Although pathogen-contaminated water is clearly a prime source of infection, it is also true that a simple insufficiency of water will hamper efforts to practise good personal and food hygiene and contribute to the transmission of disease.

Recognition of the pressing need to provide safe drinking water led to the period 1981–1990 being declared the International Drinking Water Supply and Sanitation Decade. This resulted in the WHO Guidelines for Drinking Water Quality. These guidelines place their primary emphasis on microbiological safety, though chemical contaminants can also be a problem, since more than half of the world's population is still exposed to water contaminated with pathogens.

Pests and pets

It is not just food animals that frequently carry pathogenic organisms in their gastrointestinal tract. Surveys have shown that up to 15% of pet dogs excrete salmonellae. Rats and mice can transmit illness by contaminating food with organisms picked up from sewers, garbage and other sources via their fur, urine, faeces or saliva.

Wild birds can often find their way into food processing areas, particularly in hot climates where buildings are relatively open, and these may excrete pathogens such as *Salmonella* and *Campylobacter*.

Flies, cockroaches, ants and other insect pests can transfer organisms from sources contaminated with pathogens to foods. Flies are particularly important in this respect as they are associated with both food handling areas and contaminated areas such as toilets and refuse heaps. They also have the unfortunate habit of feeding by regurgitating their previous meals on to foods to help liquefy them.

Spiders and wasps are rather less of a hazard because they tend not to breed in contaminated areas but nonetheless they have the potential to transfer pathogens to food.

The food handler

Handling of food can introduce and spread pathogenic microorganisms. Food handlers may carry pathogens without experiencing any serious ill-effects themselves. *Staphylococcus aureus* is commonly associated with the skin, nose, throat and infected skin lesions, particularly in higher primates such as humans where 20–50% of healthy individuals can carry the organism. The organism is difficult to remove from the skin where it "hides" in pores and hair follicles. If the hands are damp it can be drawn to the surface and transferred to foods. It is possible to identify carriers by microbiological testing and this has been done on a number of occasions. In one recent example, restaurant workers in Kuwait city were tested and in a sample of 500 people 26.6% were found to carry the organism (15). It is not usually feasible to do this routinely to identify *Staphylococcus aureus* carriers so, as a general precautionary measure, people should avoid handling foods with bare hands as much as possible, particularly those foods that support the growth of *S. aureus*.

Organisms that reside in the gut can be transferred to food if food handlers fail to wash their hands thoroughly after using the toilet. Gut organisms adhere less strongly to the skin and should be readily removed by washing with soap and water. Thorough hand-washing is essential after using the toilet, not just after defecation, since pathogens can also be picked up from previous users of the toilet via door handles, taps and drying towels.

The risk is very much greater if the food handler is suffering from a gut infection. In many cases, however, infected food handlers may not know that they are carrying the pathogen in their gut as they may not feel unwell and may exhibit no symptoms. This could be because they are in what is known as an acute carrier state where they are infected, can spread the organism, but have not yet begun to display symptoms. Alternatively, they may be chronic carriers who are infected but will not develop symptoms, yet will excrete the pathogen over a long period. This latter state has been most famously associated with typhoid fever, particularly the notorious case of "Typhoid Mary", a food handler who was also a chronic carrier of the illness. In the early years of the 20th century the unfortunate combination of her medical condition and her chosen profession, a cook, is estimated to have resulted in about 1300 cases of typhoid fever in the USA. Infected food handlers are also a common source of foodborne viruses such as the Hepatitis A virus and the diarrhoea-causing, small round-structured viruses which are excreted in large numbers (10^8-10^{10} g^{-1} faeces) by infected individuals. Many cases of foodborne virus infection have been associated with catering.

Equipment, utensils and kitchen practices

The equipment and utensils used in the preparation of food can also act as sources of contamination. For instance, knives or chopping boards used with uncooked products such as raw meat or poultry can become contaminated with pathogens. If they are used again without being adequately cleaned, particularly if they are then used with a cooked or ready-to-eat product, the pathogens can be transferred, posing a very serious threat to food safety. This can also happen if food handlers who work with raw food fail to wash their hands before handling ready-to-eat food. This process, whether mediated by hands or equipment, is known as cross-contamination.

Raw foods can also contaminate cooked or ready-to-eat foods if they are stored together improperly. For example, if raw meat is stored above cooked foods in a refrigerator, liquid drip from the meat can contaminate the foods stored below.

Dishcloths left wet can also act as an important reservoir of contaminating organisms that can be spread around foods and food contact surfaces as the cloth is used.

Growth

We have already noted that an important feature of the transmission of foodborne illness is that bacterial pathogens can grow in some foods. In a relatively short period, they can multiply from a low, possibly harmless level to numbers sufficient to cause illness. This does not happen with other foodborne pathogens such as parasites and viruses and it is therefore important to understand the factors that influence whether and how quickly bacteria can grow in food.

Bacteria multiply by a process of doubling; each cell splits into two identical daughter cells which go on to repeat the process, giving four cells, which then produce eight cells, and so on. The period between cell divisions is known as the generation or doubling time. This can be quite short, typically around 20 minutes or so, and sometimes even shorter. A figure of just over seven minutes at 41°C has been reported for the pathogen *Clostridium perfringens*. This means that, given the right conditions, a bacterium can multiply very rapidly from extremely low levels to numbers well in excess of the infectious doses quoted in Table 1.6. In eight hours a single organism with a generation time of 20 minutes can reach a population of more than 16 million (Figure 3.3). The ability of bacterial pathogens to multiply in foods explains why, in some circumstances, foods can be more likely to provide the minimum infective dose of a pathogen than contaminated water.

Moulds and yeasts also have the capacity to grow in foods but, with the notable exception of mycotoxin production by some moulds, this normally results in spoilage rather than health problems. Moulds and yeasts grow by different mechanisms than bacteria: most yeasts tend to multiply by budding to produce a daughter cell which separates from its parent, while moulds tend to grow as fine thread-like structures called hyphae which extend and branch to produce a tangled mass known as a mycelium.

For microorganisms to grow at their fastest, conditions have to be just right. Optimum growth conditions differ slightly for bacteria, yeasts and moulds and this can determine the type of organism that

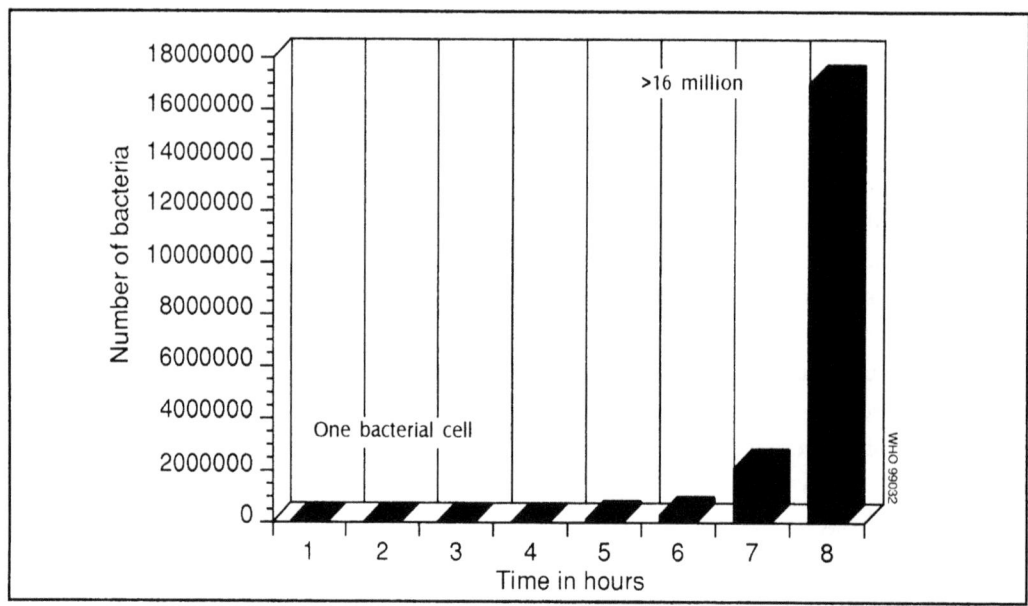

Figure 3.3 *Exponential growth of bacteria*

predominates when foods spoil. Moulds and yeasts generally grow more slowly than bacteria and are often outgrown by them unless conditions in the food are sufficiently inhibitory to bacterial growth to give the moulds and yeast a competitive advantage. The most important of the factors that affect microbial growth are:

- availability of nutrients
- temperature
- acidity/pH
- available water (water activity, a_w)
- oxygen (air)
- antimicrobial agents.
- time.

Availability of nutrients

When microorganisms grow on foods, they use them exactly as we do — as a source of nutrients and energy. Foods generally contain a variety of chemicals that serve these purposes very well and levels of nutrients are not usually limiting factors on microbial growth in foods. This means that food handling equipment must be very thoroughly cleaned after use to remove all traces of food since bacteria will grow on the tiniest remnant and this can contaminate subsequent batches.

A raw food will contain a diverse microbial population with many different organisms competing for the nutrients available. If a pathogen is present it may not do well in this competition; its supply of nutrients will be limited and it will grow only slowly or perhaps not at all. If, however, the pathogen is introduced after the food has been cooked and the natural microflora has been eliminated or severely reduced there will be little or no competition for growth and the pathogens will grow more quickly.

Pathogen growth is much less likely to occur in water where the nutrient supply is more limited.

Temperature

Microorganisms can be found growing at temperatures ranging from about -10°C up to more than 100°C. The most important consideration is that water should be present in its liquid state. If it is present either entirely in the solid state, as ice, or as water vapour, then bacteria cannot grow even if they can cope with the extreme temperature under those conditions.

Individual microorganisms will not grow over such a wide temperature span and are normally restricted to a range of about 35°C. They have a minimum temperature below which they cannot grow, a maximum temperature above which they cannot grow and in-between an optimum at which they grow best. These three temperatures, known as an organism's cardinal temperatures, are used to separate microorganisms into different classes (Table 3.1).

Table 3.1 *Cardinal temperatures for microbial growth*

Group	Temperature (°C)		
	Minimum	Optimum	Maximum
Thermophiles	40–45	55–75	60–90
Mesophiles	5–15	30–45	35–47
Psychrophiles (obligate psychrophiles)	-5–+5	12–15	15–20
Psychrotrophs (facultative psychrophiles)	-5–+5	25–30	30–35

Adapted from ICMSF, Microbial Ecology of Foods Volume 1, New York Academic Press 1980

Most foodborne pathogens are mesophiles with an optimum growth temperature around body temperature of 37°C. This makes sense since for many of them the preferred habitat is the human or animal body. In tropical developing countries foods may be stored at temperatures as high as 37°C. Mesophiles will grow rapidly at this temperature, though they can also grow quite well down to below 20°C. Their minimum growth temperature is generally around 8°C, so if a food is stored below 10°C then mesophiles will either grow very slowly or not at all (although they may *survive*, see Figure 3.4 and below).

Because of the great use of refrigeration in modern food processing, handling and distribution, there has been a lot of concern about pathogens that are capable of growing at chill temperatures (<8°C). These are the psychrotrophic pathogens (Table 3.2). Although these organisms are capable of growing in refrigerated foods, they grow very slowly. Their generation time at 4–5°C is normally 10–25 hours.

Table 3.2 Psychrotrophic foodborne pathogens

Aeromonas hydrophila
Clostridium botulinum (non-proteolytic)
Listeria monocytogenes
Yersinia enterocolitica

Freezing of foods starts at temperatures just below 0°C but is not complete until much lower temperatures are reached. Very few microorganisms will grow at temperatures below 0°C and none will grow in properly frozen foods (<-18°C) although, like microorganisms in chilled foods, they may survive and can resume growth if the temperature increases (Figure 3.4). Parasites such as protozoa, cestodes, trematodes and nematodes are much more sensitive to freezing and die during frozen storage.

No pathogenic bacteria will grow at temperatures above about 60°C and this defines the upper limit of a "danger zone" of temperature ranging from below 10°C to 60°C. Foods that are ready to serve should not be stored at temperatures in this range as there is the potential for bacterial growth to occur.

Acidity/pH

Acidity and alkalinity are measured by pH, a number which reflects the concentration of hydrogen ions present. Pure water is taken as neutral with a pH of 7. Below a pH of 7 the concentration of hydrogen ions is higher and conditions are said to be acidic; above 7, the concentration of hydrogen ions decreases and conditions are described as alkaline.

As with temperature, microorganisms will grow over a restricted range of pH and have a smaller pH range over which they grow fastest. For most bacteria the optimum pH is around neutrality (pH 7); yeasts and moulds generally have an optimum more on the acid side (below 7).

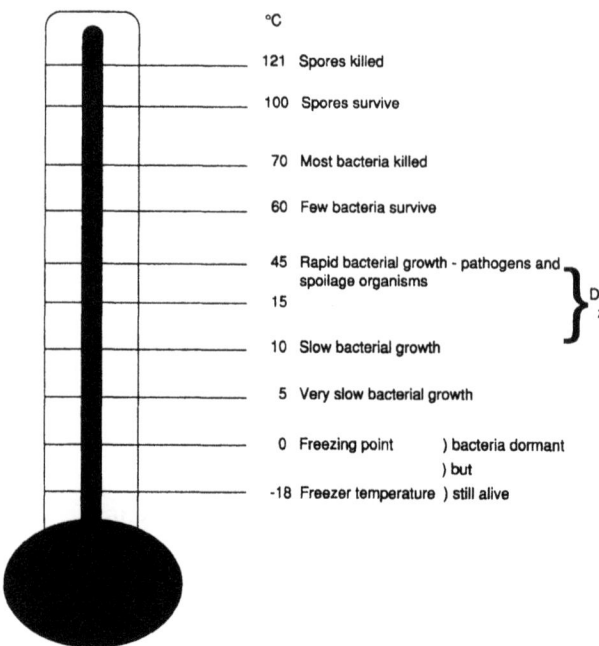

Figure 3.4 *Effect of temperature on bacterial growth*

Most foods are slightly acid although some, such as citrus fruits, pickles and sauces, are much more acidic. Pathogens cannot grow in the more acidic foods but are relatively unaffected by the pH found in most food materials. Acids differ in their ability to prevent microbial growth; acetic (ethanoic) acid is generally more effective than lactic acid which in turn is more effective than citric acid. Usually if a food has a pH below 4.5 it is considered safe from bacterial pathogens. Despite this, there have been occasional well-documented outbreaks of foodborne illness associated with acidic foods such as yoghurt.

Water activity (a_w)

All microorganisms require liquid water to enable them to grow. If there is little water present, or the water that is present is not available to the microbe, then its growth is slowed or even prevented. It may be the case that there is simply not enough water present, as in some dried foods. Alternatively, water may be present but unavailable, as in foods that contain high levels of salt or sugar and where much of the water may be "occupied" with keeping the salt or sugar in solution, or in frozen foods where the water is present as ice.

Water availability is often measured or expressed in terms of water activity (a_w). This is a scale from 0 to 1; pure water with maximum water availability has an a_w of 1, in the complete absence of water the a_w would be 0. Dried milk powder has a water activity of 0.2. Bacteria normally require a very high water availability to be able to grow at their fastest, but will often be able to grow somewhat more slowly in salty or partially dried foods. *Salmonella* will grow in the presence of 6% salt, *Listeria monocytogenes* in 10% salt, and some strains of *Staphylococcus aureus* in 20% salt. To be certain that pathogen growth is prevented, it is necessary to dry foods down to very low moisture content or add very high levels of salt or sugar (Figure 3.5). Total inhibition of growth, however, is not always necessary; *Staph. aureus* is the pathogen that is most tolerant of low water availability and will grow down to an a_w of 0.83 but it will not produce toxin if the a_w is 0.86 or below.

	Water Activity (a_w)	Food	Microorganisms & minimum a_w for growth
High moisture	1.00–0.98	Meat, fruit, milk, vegetables	
	0.98–0.95	Yogurt, evaporated milk, tomato paste	
	0.95–0.94	Baked goods	Clostridium botulinum
	0.93		Salmonella
	0.90		Most bacteria
	0.90		
	0.88–0.85	Jam, old cheese	Most yeasts, Staphylococcus aureus
	0.80		
	0.80		
	0.75	Figs, dried dates, molasses	Most moulds, halophilic
	0.70		bacteria (salt loving)
	0.70		
		Parmesan cheese, dried fruits	Osmophilic yeasts,
	0.61		xerophilic moulds
	0.60	Chocolate confectionary,	
	0.50	honey, cocoa	
	0.40	Potato flakes, crisps	
	0.30	Crackers, cake mix	
Dry	0.20	Dried milk, dried vegetables	

Figure 3.5 *Water activity, foods and microbial growth*

As a_w is decreased, bacteria are inhibited first (Figure 3.5), followed by moulds and yeasts. Some organisms are particularly adapted to growing at low a_w values — such as the halophilic bacteria, and some moulds and yeasts — but these are associated mainly with spoilage problems. No microbial growth at all occurs when the a_w is below 0.6.

The a_w of a food is also related to the relative humidity of its storage environment. If a food is stored in a closed container and allowed to equilibrate with the atmosphere that surrounds it, the relative humidity of the atmosphere will become equal to the a_w of the food. Thus, for example, dried fruit with an a_w of 0.72 would be in equilibrium with an atmospheric relative humidity of 72% (0.72 of saturation). This has important implications for the storage of dried foods where, if the relative humidity of the environment is higher than the a_w, water will condense on the food. This will increase the food's a_w, perhaps bringing it into a range where mould growth can occur.

Oxygen (air)

Air comprises about 20% oxygen. Most microorganisms grow much faster if oxygen is present at this concentration and are known as aerobes. Some, such as moulds, are obligate aerobes which means that they cannot grow at all if air (oxygen) is absent. However, for some bacteria — the obligate anaerobes — the presence of oxygen is actually toxic. Restricting the presence of oxygen and increasing the level of other gases such as carbon dioxide is a useful way of preserving some foods since many of the normal spoilage organisms will not grow under these conditions. Pathogenic bacteria, however, are largely unaffected. Most are what are known as facultative anaerobes which can grow in the presence or absence of air, and some, such as *Clostridium botulinum* and *Clostridium perfringens*, are obligate anaerobes and positively require oxygen-free conditions.

Antimicrobial agents

Foods were all once living organisms which possessed systems to protect them from microbial infections that might damage them. Some of these systems can persist into the food product and help inhibit microbial growth. They are mainly associated with plant foods, though there are a number of antimicrobial systems in foods such as eggs and milk that contribute to their stability. Some antimicrobial plant components such as benzoic acid have also been deliberately added to foods as preservatives. Generally their effect is limited and should not be overestimated. Garlic when crushed produces the antimicrobial component, allicin, but crushed garlic in oil has nevertheless been the cause of a botulism outbreak (*16*).

Antimicrobials are added to foods principally to inhibit spoilage organisms. One notable exception to this is the artificial preservative nitrite which is of major importance in cured meats as an inhibitor of *Clostridium botulinum*. Outbreaks of botulism caused by cured meats are often the result of failures in the curing process which have resulted in insufficient nitrite being present.

Time

The final, and in many ways the most important factor of all, is time. Bacteria can grow to dangerous levels if they have the right conditions for growth, but only if they have sufficient time to do so. Microorganisms will grow fastest in foods with no inhibitory factors and these therefore have the shortest safe shelf-life. However, a food may have a water availability and pH that slows the growth of a pathogen but this will be of little help if the food is left for long periods allowing sufficient growth to occur.

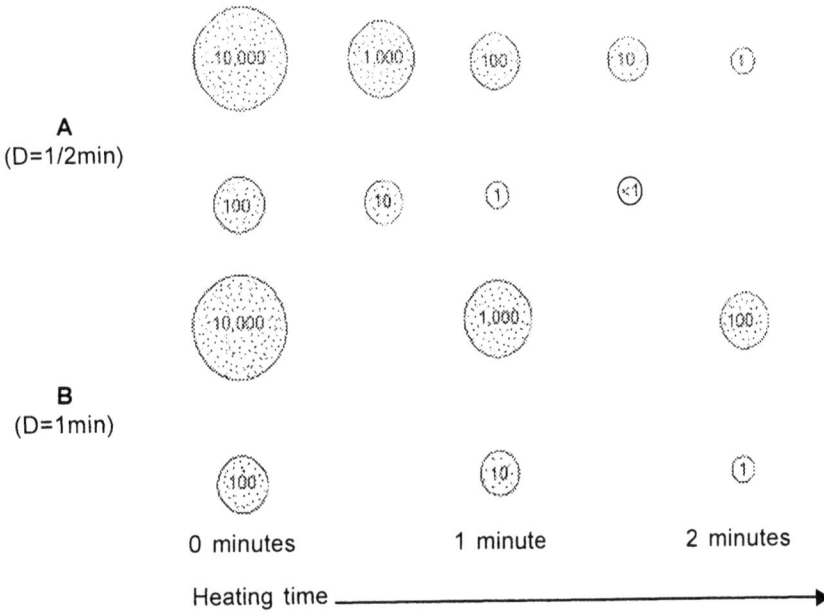

Figure 3.6 *Effect of heat resistance (D value) and initial numbers on the survival of bacteria during heating*

Survival

It is also important not to forget the possibility of microbial survival. If bacteria are present in sufficient numbers in a food, it may not be necessary for them to *grow* in it to produce illness; all they have to do is *survive* to maintain those numbers. This is well illustrated by the bacterial pathogen *Campylobacter jejuni* which does not normally grow in foods but has a low infectious dose and can survive to cause illness. Viruses will multiply only in the cells of the infected individual but can survive in, and be transmitted by, foods.

The question of bacterial survival is particularly important since, in many cases, conditions that prevent growth enhance survival. For example, microorganisms cannot grow in dried foods and frozen foods, but they can survive in these foods for very long periods with only a slight decrease in numbers. Foods which will not support microbial growth can still, therefore, contain pathogenic bacteria in numbers sufficient to cause illness. Even where the numbers are low, the bacteria present can resume growth and multiply very rapidly to high levels if conditions are changed. This could happen if, for example, a dehydrated product is mixed with water and left to stand, or a frozen food is left too long defrosting at temperatures suitable for pathogen growth.

Some adverse conditions do affect both microbial growth and survival. If the pH is too low for a microorganism to grow, it will die slowly during storage. It may, however, take some time for the food to become safe. Little is currently known about the survival of non-bacterial pathogens such as viruses and parasites at the pH levels normally found in foods.

The most effective and accessible way of killing microorganisms is by heating. Above the maximum temperature which supports their growth, microorganisms will die. The rate at which they die will increase as the temperature increases. The conventional way in which we describe

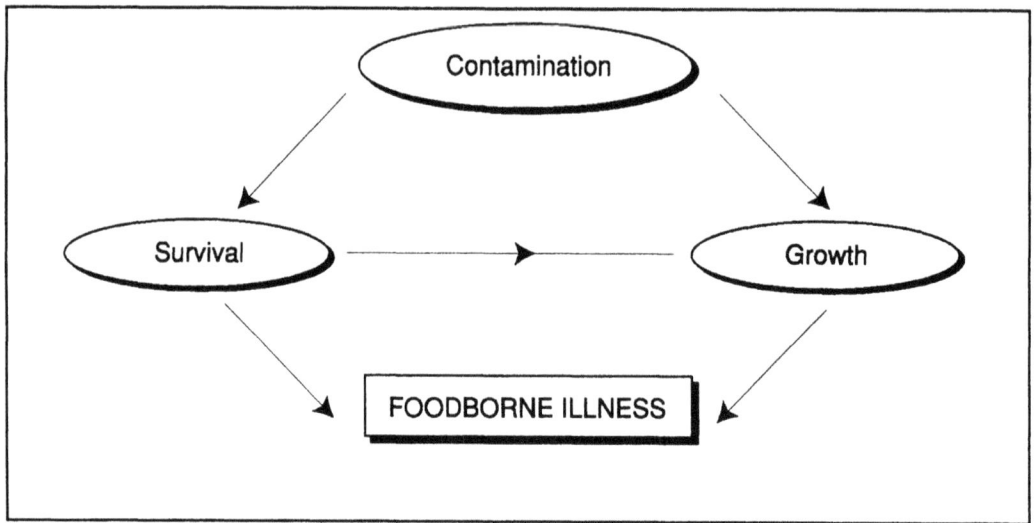

Figure 3.7 *Factors leading to foodborne illness*

this rate is by what is known as a D-value. The D-value for an organism is the time that it takes at a particular temperature to kill 90% of a population of that organism, i.e. to reduce the number of viable cells by a factor of 10. The smaller the D-value, the faster the death rate at that temperature.

Measured D-values are quite variable and depend on the type of food material and the particular strain of the organism concerned, but for a high moisture product a typical bacterial D-value at 65°C can be 0.1–0.5 minutes (6–30 seconds). If the temperature is increased by about 5°C then the death rate will increase about 10-fold.

How long a food needs to be heated to make it safe also depends on how many organisms are present initially (Figure 3.6). High numbers will take longer to kill. To predict accurately how long a food should be heated and at what temperature requires quite a detailed knowledge of the food and the pathogens present but, as a general rule, a food should be cooked so that all of it reaches at least 70°C.

Cooking is not just a useful procedure to eliminate foodborne bacteria. Foodborne viruses and parasites can also be killed, although in these cases we do not have such detailed knowledge of their thermal stability. Foodborne toxins, however, may be unaffected by heating. Most mycotoxins are stable to normal cooking procedures, as are some bacterial toxins such as those produced by *Staphylococcus aureus* and *Bacillus cereus*.

Some pathogenic bacteria such as *Clostridium perfringens*, *Clostridium botulinum* and *Bacillus cereus* produce heat-resistant spores. These will not be killed by conventional cooking procedures and could resume growth after cooking if the food is stored for too long at an inappropriate temperature.

The ability of cooking to solve food safety problems is not therefore unlimited and wherever possible prevention of dangerous levels of contamination in the first place is preferable.

Foods processed commercially which have received a moderate heat treatment specifically designed to eliminate non-spore forming pathogens and/or spoilage bacteria are described as being pasteurized. To eliminate sporeforming pathogens and spoilage organisms heat processes far in excess of normal cooking, sometimes known as appertization, are necessary. This is the treatment given to canned foods to ensure that they can be stored safely for long periods without re-

Table 3.3 Factors contributing to outbreaks of foodborne illness

	England and Wales[1]	U.S.A.[2]
Preparation too far in advance	57	29
Storage at ambient temperature	38	63
Inadequate cooling	32	
Contaminated processed food	17	n.i.
Undercooking	15	5
Contaminated canned food	7	n.i.
Inadequate thawing	6	n.i.
Cross contamination	6	15
Food consumed raw	6	n.i.
Improper warm handling	5	27
Infected food handlers	4	26
Use of left overs	4	7
Extra large quantities prepared	3	n.i.

1. 1320 outbreaks between 1970 and 1982 from Roberts 1985.
2. Outbreaks occurring between 1973 and 1976 from Bryan 1978.
   n.i. category not included in analysis.

frigeration. Further reference to these two processes is made in Chapter 5.

Treatment of food with ionizing radiation is similar to heat in its effect on microorganisms. Non-sporeforming bacteria and parasites will be killed by quite low doses (less than 10 kGy). This can be considered the radiation equivalent of pasteurization and is termed *radicidation*. Bacterial spores and viruses are more resistant and require much higher doses to ensure their elimination. Such doses can often produce unacceptable flavour changes in the product and are less likely to be used in normal commercial practice.

Major factors leading to foodborne illness

We have looked at the three factors that contribute to the presence of dangerous numbers of microorganisms in a food — contamination, growth, and survival (Figure 3.7).

Hygienic food handling aims to control the presence of pathogens in foods by controlling each of these contributory factors. When outbreaks of foodborne illness occur it is because there has been a loss of control over one of these factors.

WHO data indicate that only a small number of factors related to food handling are responsible for a large proportion of foodborne disease episodes everywhere. Common errors include:

- preparation of food several hours prior to consumption, combined with its storage at temperatures which favour the growth of pathogenic bacteria or the formation of toxins;

- insufficient cooking or reheating of food to reduce or eliminate pathogens;

- cross-contamination;
- people with poor personal hygiene handling the food.

There have been several studies of outbreaks of foodborne illness which attempt to identify where the failure has occurred. The results of two such surveys are shown in Table 3.3.

Two points should be apparent from this table. Firstly, the percentages in each column do not add up to 100%. This reflects the fact that in many outbreaks several failures of good hygienic practices were identified. This is perhaps not so surprising since, if people are not familiar with what good practices are, they are likely to make more than just one error. It may also reflect the fact that to achieve an infective dose of a pathogen can require a combination of several errors: initial contamination with the pathogen, allowing it to multiply, and then failing to eliminate it by adequate cooking. The second significant point is that the most commonly identified causes are failure to control temperature and time — failure to cool foods correctly and store them at temperatures that prevent microbial growth, failure to heat them sufficiently to kill microorganisms, or prolonged storage giving microorganisms time to multiply to dangerous levels.

KEY POINTS

- Microorganisms are everywhere.

- Microorganisms can cause illness, they can spoil food, and some can ferment it into desired products.

- Pathogenic microorganisms can be part of a food's natural microflora, or may be contaminants.

- Contaminants can come from the normal environment, a polluted environment, pests and pets, the food handler and/or equipment.

- Bacteria and moulds are able to grow in foods, increasing the risks that they pose.

- The growth of bacteria and moulds can be extremely rapid.

- This growth is affected by the composition of the food and its storage environment.

- The possibilities of both *growth* and *survival* of bacteria must be considered when assessing safety.

- Heating is the most effective single method for improving food safety.

- Ionizing radiation can also help make food safe.

- A number of different factors contribute to outbreaks of foodborne illness, but most include a failure to control temperature/time.

Chapter 4
Hazards associated with different foods and their control

Red meat, poultry and their products

Meat can be derived from a huge variety of birds, mammals and reptiles, though cattle, sheep, goats, pigs and poultry (chickens, ducks, turkeys) are the principal sources. In many countries, meat is also the product that is most often associated with problems of microbiological food safety. There are two main reasons for this:

- Fresh meat provides bacteria with an ideal medium on which they can grow. It has ample nutrients, available water and a moderate pH.

- The animal or bird can also act as the source of pathogenic organisms such as bacteria and parasites found in meat. It acquires these from its environment, feed, water or other animals. As outlined in Chapter 3, the skin and gastrointestinal tract of the healthy animal carry a large population of microorganisms that can include a number of pathogenic bacteria such as *Escherichia coli*, *Salmonella* and *Campylobacter*. These come primarily from the animal's gut but can be transferred to the skin via faeces. Parasites, if present, can be found at a number of locations in the animal's body.

A first step towards ensuring good quality meat is, of course, to exclude the use of meat from obviously diseased or sick animals and to inspect carcasses for signs of parasitic infections. Good microbiological quality meat, however, also depends on hygienic slaughter and butchering — avoiding the contamination of freshly exposed meat surfaces from the hide or contents of the gut, either directly or via the workers' hands, clothing, equipment or via pests such as flies.

Good hygienic practices in this area can reduce contamination but do not necessarily guarantee freedom from pathogenic microorganisms. Raw meat should therefore always be regarded as a likely source of pathogens. This is supported by statistics from various countries. For example, in the United Kingdom meat or poultry dishes were incriminated in more than 74% of incidents of foodborne illness.

Most meat products are cooked before consumption and this eliminates the vegetative forms of bacteria as well as viruses and parasites. With intact pieces of meat, most of the microorganisms will be associated with the meat surfaces and will be readily killed by heat. However, if the meat has been comminuted, microorganisms will be mixed into the bulk of the meat making it more hazardous unless thoroughly cooked throughout. Serious recent outbreaks of illness caused by *E. coli* O157 have been linked with the failure to cook ground or minced meat products adequately.

Cooking is therefore an important measure for ensuring that food is safe, though on its own it is not always sufficient. Microbial growth before cooking must be controlled as far as possible to prevent the production of heat stable toxins such as those of *Staphylococcus aureus*. Heat-resistant bacterial endospores of *Clostridium perfringens* and other sporeformers are resistant to temperatures above 100°C and will survive normal cooking. If the meat is not adequately cooled after cooking the spores may germinate, the organisms may grow and may rapidly produce large numbers of vegetative cells. If the cooked meat is then eaten cold or not adequately reheated before consumption to destroy the vegetative cells, illness will probably result. Precooked meat dishes such as joints, stews and casseroles are very common vehicles for this type of foodborne illness. In some cases, however, the meat may not be the source of the organism. In many countries it is common practice to add a range of spices and herbs to cooked meat dishes and these may be the source of the *Clostridium perfringens* spores. For example, one study found a greater incidence of *Clostridium perfringens* in foods in Pakistan than in Zambia and this difference was attributed to the greater culinary use of spices in Pakistan.

If spices or herbs are added after cooking when the food has cooled slightly, there is also the opportunity for non-sporeforming pathogens such as *Salmonella* or *Shigella* to survive and grow in the product if they are present on the added ingredient.

Cooked meats served cold can be particularly hazardous. They are susceptible to contamination from uncooked products which can reintroduce many of the organisms killed by cooking. They may also be subject to environmental contamination with organisms such as *Listeria monocytogenes*, and handling can introduce *Staphylococcus aureus*. Both of these bacteria grow well in meats and can also grow readily at the salt levels normally found in cured cooked meats. Contaminants introduced into cooked meats even at quite low levels could pose a serious threat since they may grow even more rapidly than usual as cooking will have reduced competition from other bacteria. The absence of further cooking also means that the viable organisms will persist in the product until it is consumed.

A number of meat products contain additives such as nitrite and, in some countries, sulfur dioxide. Nitrite is particularly important in the control of *Clostridium botulinum* in cured meats such as hams and sausages and failure to cure meats sufficiently has resulted in occasional outbreaks of botulism. Because of the distinctive symptoms, such outbreaks can be traced back hundreds of years. This long association of botulism with such meat products is also reflected in the name of the organism which is derived from *botulus*, the Latin word for sausage.

Sulfur dioxide is used in some countries as a meat preservative, where its principal purpose is to delay spoilage. In doing so it inhibits mainly Gram-negative bacteria which include many important pathogens such as *Salmonella*.

As a general rule it is not advisable to eat uncooked meat and this rule is generally adhered to (popular raw meat dishes such as steak tartare being a notable exception). Many fermented sausages such as salamis are, however, also essentially raw meat products. Most receive no heat treatment during their processing and rely on a combination of antibacterial factors or hurdles for their keeping quality and safety. They are cured products containing a mixture of salt (sodium chloride) and nitrite, both of which will inhibit bacterial growth. They are also dried to various extents, depending on the product, and undergo a fermentation by lactic acid bacteria which converts sugar to lactic acid, decreasing the pH. If the product is well made, using good quality meat and an efficient starter culture to ensure a rapid lactic fermentation and pH drop, it is unlikely to pose a problem. In such cases, the presence of pathogens in the raw material would be very low and those that might be present would have little opportunity to grow and would be likely to die during processing. Failure to observe these rules can, and has, resulted in outbreaks of illness caused by *Salmonella* and *Staphylococcus aureus*.

Eggs and egg products

Eggs are an animal product with a long association with *Salmonella*. Normally contamination is located on the outside of the shell as a result of contact with the hen's faeces in the cloaca or in the nest after laying. The egg shell is normally an excellent barrier for preventing bacterial penetration of the egg. Penetration can occur, however, under conditions of high temperature and humidity, and more commonly with duck eggs than with hens' eggs. Some *Salmonella* serotypes are particularly host-adapted and can infect egg yolk in the oviduct. In hens' eggs, this has been associated in recent years with certain types of *Salmonella enteritidis*.

Salmonella adhering to the outside of the shell with faecal material may contaminate the contents once the egg is broken. This can be a problem since eggs are often lightly cooked and are not cooked at all in a number of foods where they are used for their functional properties. This type of contamination is most likely to occur when large numbers of eggs are broken in commercial food processing and, for this reason, bulk liquid egg is pasteurized (generally at 64.5°C for 2½ minutes). It may also occur at household level, if care is not taken when breaking eggs, and this has been the cause of a number of outbreaks of salmonellosis.

Milk and dairy products

Milk carefully drawn from the healthy animal will have very low levels of bacterial contaminants. However, in practice this milk rapidly acquires microorganisms from the animal, its immediate environment and from equipment. Some of these microorganisms could be pathogens, a number of which are associated with raw milk (Table 4.1).

Table 4.1 Examples of pathogens associated with milk

Mycobacterium bovis
Brucella spp.
Salmonella
Campylobacter
Listeria monocytogenes
E. coli
Yersinia enterocolitica
Staphylococcus aureus
Bacillus cereus

In many countries it is required to heat-treat milk before sale to destroy pathogens that may be present. Several possible combinations of temperature and time are often specified in regulations that

Table 4.2 *Examples of time-temperature heat treatment for pasteurization of milk*

Low temperature holding (LTH)	63 °C for 30 minutes
High temperature short time (HTST)	72 °C for 15 seconds
Ultra high temperature (UHT)	135 °C for 1 second
"Sterilised"	>100 °C typically 20–40 minutes

must be followed carefully (Table 4.2). It is possible to test milk to see if it has been adequately heat-treated. Raw milk contains an enzyme, phosphatase, that is inactivated by the prescribed heat treatments. In the test, a chemical is added to a sample of milk which the enzyme, if present, will convert to a bright yellow compound. Failure to observe a yellow colour therefore indicates that the enzyme is not active and that the milk has been correctly pasteurized.

Where commercially heat-processed milk is not widely available, it is both common practice and a wise precaution to boil milk before it is consumed.

Heat processing will destroy all but the heat-resistant spores such as those of *Bacillus cereus*. *B. cereus* is a common spoilage organism of heat-treated milks, but milk-associated cases of *B. cereus* intoxication are rare. Heating will also not destroy the enterotoxin produced by *Staphylococcus aureus* and outbreaks have been caused by dried milk where *S. aureus* was allowed to grow and produce enterotoxin before drying.

Inadequate pasteurization or environmental contamination of milk with *Salmonella* after pasteurization has also caused problems with dried milk. Under dry conditions, the organism can survive for prolonged periods though it cannot grow until the milk is rehydrated. Extremely high standards of hygiene are therefore essential in the processing of milk.

Most commercial processing of milk into products such as cheese, yoghurt, butter and dried milks includes a preliminary pasteurization or equivalent heat treatment to assure their safety. Many traditional milk products such as cheeses, butter and yoghurts, however, evolved before the advent of pasteurization because they were safer and more stable than raw milk. A number of factors contribute to this: yoghurt has a low pH and hard cheeses combine a reduced pH with a low moisture content. Butter has a special physical structure where the water is present as many tiny globules spread through a continuous fat phase. Microorganisms in these globules find it difficult to grow because of limited space and nutrients and the relatively high local concentration of salt. The antibacterial effect of these factors does not have the same degree of certainty that is associated with heat treatment. Therefore there is a greater risk of these products causing illness when they are made from raw milk since it is more likely to contain pathogens at a level sufficient for some to survive processing. This is reflected in Table 4.3 which describes reported outbreaks of foodborne illness due to cheese since 1980 and shows the preponderance of cheeses made from raw milk.

Fish, shellfish and fishery products

Fish and shellfish can become contaminated from their natural environment or from subsequent handling or processing.

Fish and shellfish act as intermediate hosts for a number of parasites that can infect humans (Table 4.4). Illness caused

Table 4.3 *Examples of reported outbreaks of foodborne disease due to cheeses*

Outbreak	Pathogen	no. of cases	no. of deaths	Food
USA, 1985	L. monocytogenes	>142	48	mexican-style cheese*
Switzerland, 1983–87	L. monocytogenes	>122	34	Vacherin Mont d'Or cheese**
France, 1995	L. monocytogenes	20	4	Brie de Meaux cheese**
Canada, 1984	Salmonella Typhimurium	2700	1	Cheddar cheese**
Switzerland, 1985	Salmonella Typhimurium	>40	0	Vacherin Mont d'Or cheese**
England, 1989	Salmonella Dublin	42	0	Irish soft cheese**
USA, 1989	Salmonella Javiana and S. Oranienberg	164	0	Mozzarella cheese
France, 1993	Salmonella Paratyphi B	273	1	goat's milk cheese**
Netherlands, Denmark, Sweden, USA, 1983	Enterotoxigenic Escherichia coli	>3000	NR	Brie cheese***
Scotland, 1994	Verotoxin-forming E.coli O157	>20#	0	local, farm-produced cheese**
Scotland, 1984–85	Staphyloccus aureus enterotoxin	>13	0	sheep milk cheese**
England, 1988–89	Suspected Staphylococcus aureus enterotoxin	155	0	Stilton cheese**
Malta, 1995	Brucella melitensis	35	1	Soft cheese**

* Pasteurised milk was used, but there was evidence that unpasteurised milk was also included.
** These products are known to have been produced using unpasteurised milk.
*** Many Brie cheese are made from unpasteurised milk.
NR: not reported.
one case of haemolytic uraemic syndrome.
Data from Food Safety and Raw Milk Cheese. Professional Food Microbiologist Group of the IFST.

Table 4.4 *Helminths transmitted to humans in seafood*

Disease	Causative organism(s)	Seafood
Small intestinal fluke infection		
Echinostomiosis	Echinostoma spp	Freshwater fishes
	Artyfechinostomum malayanum	Freshwater fishes, prawns, crabs, freshwater snails
Heterophyiosis	Heterophyes heterophyes	Brackish water
	Heterophyes spp.	Fishes, mullet
	Metagonimus yokogawai[a]	Trout
Liver fluke infection		
Clonorchiosis	Clonorchis sinensis	Freshwater fishes
Opisthorchiosis	Opisthorchis felineus	Freshwater fishes
	Opisthorchis spp.	Fishes
Lung fluke infection		
Paragonimiosis	Paragonimus westermani	Fishes, crabs, crayfish, prawns, mammals
	Paragonimus spp.	Crabs, crayfish, prawns
Broad fish tapeworm infection		
Diphyllobothriosis	Diphyllobothrium spp.	Marine and freshwater fishes
Larva migrans		
Gnathostomiosis	Gnathostoma spinigerum	Freshwater fishes, frogs, snakes, birds
	Gnathostoma spp.	Freshwater fishes
Eosinophilic meningoencephalitis		
Angiostrongyliosis	Angiostrongylus cantonenesis	Snails, fish, crabs, shrimp, frogs
Visceral larval migrans		
Angiostrongyliosis	Angiostrongylus costaricensis	Mollucs
Gastrointestinal invasion		
Anisakiasis	Anisakis spp.	Marine fishes, octopus, squid
	Pseudoterranova spp.	
	Contracaecum spp.	
	Phocascaris spp.	
Intestinal capillariosis		
Capillariosis	Capillaria philippinensis	Marine and freshwater fishes

[a] M. takahashii, H. nocens, H. dispar, Heterophyopsis continua. Pygidiopsis summa. Stellant chasmus falcatus. Centrocestus armatus and Stictodora fuscatum are known from Korea
Source: Emerging problems in seafood borne parasitic zoonoses. Food Control, 1992, 3:2–7.

by fishborne parasites has been severely under-reported in the past and its extent as a food safety problem is only just emerging. Travel and changing food habits mean that it is not a problem confined to developing countries, the incidence of anisakiasis, for instance, is increasing in the United States. Although parasites will be readily killed by thorough cooking, in many countries raw, lightly cooked or marinaded fish can be common. These preparation practices, which are being used more widely, do not guarantee elimination of parasites.

Fish from warmer coastal waters can often be contaminated with the bacterium *Vibrio parahaemolyticus* and this can be transferred to other fish both at the market and in the home. *V. parahaemolyticus* is readily killed by thorough cooking but can be spread to cooked fish by inadequate separation of raw and cooked products. *Vibrio vulnificus* is associated with seafoods, particularly oysters, which are often eaten uncooked. It does not cause diarrhoea but is responsible for very severe extra-intestinal infections such as life-threatening septicaemia in patients who normally have some other underlying disease.

Vibrio cholerae is often transmitted by water but foods that have been in contact with contaminated water or faeces from infected persons frequently also serve as a vehicle of infection. These would naturally include fish from contaminated water or washed with it after being caught. The organism would be killed by cooking but recent cases of cholera in South America have been associated with the uncooked fish marinade *ceviche*.

Water polluted with sewage is a particular problem with filter-feeding molluscan shellfish such as oysters and mussels which are often eaten raw or after only light cooking. These feed by filtering nutrients from large volumes of their surrounding water, at the same time accumulating microorganisms from their environment. Since they are mainly harvested from shallow coastal waters where sewage contamination is likely to be greatest, they are commonly contaminated with pathogenic bacteria and viruses of human (and animal) enteric origin. Numbers of pathogenic bacteria in their tissues can be reduced by transferring the shellfish to clean coastal waters (relaying) or by holding them in tanks in which the water is recirculated and disinfected with ultraviolet light (a process known as depuration). While this is an effective and well proven procedure for bacteria, it is far less so for viruses which seem to persist much longer in shellfish tissues under these conditions.

Fish can also be the cause of a number of different intoxications where cooking does not eliminate the problem. These toxins are often the products of algae. When these algae are consumed by filter-feeding shellfish or small herbivorous fish, the toxin accumulates in the flesh which may then be consumed and accumulated by larger carnivorous fish, which in turn may be eaten by humans. Ciguatera is an example of this where the toxin (ciguatoxin) is produced by the dinoflagellate alga *Gambierdiscus toxicus* and then amplified through the food chain. This particular condition occurs only with fish from tropical and subtropical regions but other types of dinoflagellate intoxication occur in cooler climates. Usually this follows an algal bloom where environmental conditions lead to a sudden proliferation of the toxin-producing algae. A number of different illnesses have been identified: paralytic shellfish poisoning caused by toxins produced by the *Alexandrium (Gonyaulax)* species and others; neurotoxic shellfish poisoning, which follows so-called red tides, caused by *Ptychodiscus brevis*; and diarrhoeic shellfish poisoning caused by toxins produced by *Dinophysis fortii* (see

Table 2.3). These types of foodborne illness are controlled by monitoring for incidents of algal blooms and banning the harvesting and sale of shellfish from the areas where they occur.

Scombrotoxic fish poisoning is an intoxication that exhibits the symptoms of histamine toxicity. Scombroid fish such as tuna, bonito and mackerel have mainly been implicated although non-scombroid fish such as sardines, pilchards and herrings have also caused cases. It is thought that bacterial decomposition of the fish flesh leads to toxin production as freshly caught fish have not been implicated. The toxin is heat stable since outbreaks have been caused by canned fish. The potential toxicity of fish is assessed by measuring the level of histamine present, although this does not appear to be the toxic agent since it has not proved possible to reproduce the symptoms in volunteers fed histamine and some cases have been reported where the fish implicated contained low levels of histamine.

Fish products can pose a number of food safety hazards when critical steps in processing are not adequately controlled. For example, cooked products must always be protected against contamination after cooking. In commercial fish products, one example where this has been a particular problem is frozen, peeled, cooked prawns, where pathogens can be introduced during the extensive handling of the product after cooking.

In many fish products, salt is an important factor in limiting the growth of pathogens. For example, pre-salting is a common practice in fish drying where it helps accelerate drying while limiting the growth of bacteria during the process. In smoked fish, a minimum salt content of 3% in the water phase and an internal temperature of at least 63°C during smoking have been recommended in order to control *Clostridium botulinum*.

Problems with *Clostridium botulinum* have been encountered with some traditional fermented fish products. These rely on a combination of salt and reduced pH for their safety. If the product has insufficient salt, or fails to achieve a rapid pH drop to below 4.5, *C. botulinum* can grow.

Fruits and vegetables

As described in Chapter 2, some fruits and vegetables can be hazardous as a result of their intrinsic toxicity. This problem is best avoided by using only those plant products with a record of safe use and by employing well established methods for safe preparation (e.g. in cassava processing).

Contamination from pesticide residues or other environmental chemicals may also pose problems. Such hazards are best controlled by using proper agricultural practices and protecting growing crops from sources of environmental contamination.

During cultivation, harvest and storage, fruits and vegetables may become contaminated with pathogens from sources such as water, soil and animal or bird excreta. The risk of such contamination can be greatly increased as a result of practices such as using manure or human sewage as a fertilizer or irrigating with sewage-polluted water. The problem is likely to be worse in those products that grow in or very near the ground. The liver fluke *Fasciola hepatica* has been transmitted via watercress as a result of contamination of the growing beds with cattle or sheep manure.

Species of *Bacillus*, *Clostridium* and *Listeria monocytogenes* can all be introduced from the soil, while the full range of enteric pathogens spread by the faecal-oral route (parasites such as *Entamoeba histolytica* and

Giardia, viruses such as rotavirus, Norwalk-type agents, hepatitis A virus, and bacteria such as *Shigella, Salmonella, E. coli* and *Vibrio cholerae*) can all be introduced as a result of contamination by sewage.

Once again, cooking will eliminate all but the sporeforming bacteria and these may grow if the cooked product is stored unrefrigerated for extended periods. For example, wrapping pre-cooked potatoes or other root crops in aluminium foil creates anaerobic conditions and could lead to the growth of *Clostridium botulinum*.

Contamination on fruits and vegetables that are eaten without cooking can be reduced by washing them thoroughly with clean water. Inclusion of a disinfecting agent such as hypochlorite in the water can improve the elimination of microorganisms associated with the product but this does not guarantee safety. The surface of many fruits and vegetables is not smooth and has many small indentations where microorganisms may "hide", remaining on the product even after quite extensive washing. If the water used to wash fruit or vegetables is contaminated, this can, of course, have precisely the opposite effect and introduce dangerous contamination.

Microbial growth on intact fruits or vegetables will be limited because the plant possesses natural antimicrobial barriers in the form of the skin, shell or rind which protect it from infection during life. The plant surface is a relatively inhospitable environment for most pathogens and they will not be able to grow, though they may survive. Any damage that breaches these antimicrobial layers will lead to microbial invasion and growth in the underlying tissues, so any form of processing such as chopping, slicing or peeling will increase potential for the growth or survival of contaminants and the risk of transmission of foodborne illness. This is a food safety problem mainly in the case of vegetables because their tissues are less acidic than those of fruits. It is a particular concern in the commercial production of pre-prepared salad vegetables which are more extensively handled and processed than most other products. This means that great care has to be taken in the sourcing and hygienic processing of ingredients. In acidic products like citrus fruits, the pH is generally too low to support the growth of pathogens and damage simply results in spoilage by more acid-tolerant organisms such as yeasts and moulds. Pathogens can, however, survive on the outer surfaces of these products.

Mouldy products will already have had their antimicrobial barriers breached. This can lead to bacterial growth but can also result in contamination with mycotoxins produced by moulds. Mycotoxins are mainly associated with products such as cereals and oilseeds but contamination of fruit and vegetables is also known. The mycotoxin patulin produced by several species of *Penicillium* is most often associated with moulded apples. It can also contaminate juices made from moulded fruit. Toxigenic strains of the species *Fusarium* have been isolated from bananas and the mycotoxins diacetoxyscirpenol and zearalenone have sometimes been detected at very high levels. Aflatoxin contamination has also been found on occasion in dried fruits such as raisins and figs.

Mould infestation does not always indicate contamination with mycotoxins, and conversely mycotoxins can sometimes be present in a product in the absence of any obvious moulding. As a general precautionary measure, obviously mouldy foods should be avoided.

Traditional forms of processing such as pickling and fermentation rely on acidic conditions to ensure the safety and keeping quality of a food product. At low pH, pathogens will not grow and will die during storage. Procedures such as drying will not remove pathogens though they will not grow on the dried product. Sun-drying could, however, result in the introduction of pathogens through contamination from birds, flies or rodents.

Cereals and cereal products

Mycotoxins are the main food safety hazard associated with cereals and their products. Cereals can be infected with mycotoxigenic moulds, sometimes in the field, but more commonly during improper storage. These toxins can persist through processing into the final food product.

Bacteria are less of a direct threat since the low moisture content of cereals during storage prevents their growth. Organisms such as *Salmonella* may occasionally be present as a result of faecal contamination but the bacteria most commonly found surviving on cereals and their flours are species of the sporeformer *Bacillus*.

Cereal products are nearly always cooked before consumption to gelatinize the starch and make them more palatable and digestible. This will also eliminate the non-sporeformers from the product. If the cooked product has a sufficiently high water activity and is stored at an appropriate temperature, the spores of *Bacillus cereus* and other toxigenic *Bacillus* species can germinate and grow to cause illness. There is a common association of foodborne illness from *Bacillus* species with starchy products such as rice and pasta dishes, sauces thickened with cornflour and various breads.

Starchy suspensions in water make an excellent growth medium for almost any bacterial pathogen if it is introduced. A large international outbreak of illness caused by *Staphylococcus aureus* in pasta occurred when the starchy dough was contaminated with the organism and left too long, allowing growth and toxin production before drying. In many African countries, a cereal porridge is a staple food and post-cooking contamination of this has been implicated as a vehicle in the transmission of weanling diarrhoea by a number of different pathogens. In some areas these porridges traditionally undergo a lactic fermentation and there is evidence that this is a useful way of improving the safety of these products. The lactic acid and low pH in these porridges has been shown to inhibit a wide range of bacterial pathogens and one study has suggested a lower incidence of diarrhoea in children where fermented porridges are consumed (*17*).

Bottled waters

The importance of polluted water as a source of pathogenic organisms has been discussed briefly in Chapter 3 and the beneficial impact of supplies of clean safe water on public health is difficult to overstate. Bottled waters are produced throughout the world and are increasingly popular in many countries. These are generally produced from water that is completely free of pathogenic organisms. For example, natural mineral waters within the European Union must come from a specified underground source that is protected from any kind of pollution. Other types of bottled water can be produced from alternative sources, including the public water supply. The sources used naturally tend to be those that are unpolluted and this should be confirmed by microbiological analysis. After abstraction such waters can also be subjected to disinfection treatments, usually involving a combination of filtration, ozonization and irradiation with ultraviolet light. Where bottled waters are carbonated this too has a strong antimicrobial effect. As a result bottled waters have a very good health record. One notable exception to this was when bottled water was implicated as a vehicle of infection in a cholera outbreak in Portugal in 1974 (*18*).

Though the water used may be very pure microbiologically, this may not always be true of the bottles that are used. Organisms in the bottles can produce visible growth during prolonged storage of the product, though this is generally more of an acceptability problem than a health hazard. One Japanese survey of imported and home-produced bottled waters found visible microbial growth, principally mould growth, in 20% of the samples examined (*19*).

KEY POINTS

- Raw foods can contain pathogens from a variety of sources.

- Animal products are the most likely foods to contain pathogens.

- Plant products may also be contaminated with pathogens, particularly if they have been exposed to sewage or sewage-contaminated water.

- Correct processing can help control the growth/survival of pathogens.

- Cooking/heating is the most effective and reliable way of improving food safety.

- Commercially canned foods are generally safe.

- Good hygiene rules must be followed regardless of the food being processed.

Chapter 5
Technologies for the control of hazards

Some of the safety implications of food processing were introduced in Chapter 4 when discussing individual food types. However, since many food processing technologies are applied to various kinds of food, some general principles are best illustrated by considering the technologies themselves.

Food preservation technologies are intended to improve the keeping quality and safety of food commodities. In most cases this is done by influencing in some way the microorganisms that cause spoilage and foodborne illness. The technologies can be classified according to how they affect the microorganisms, namely:

- technologies that prevent contamination;

- technologies that control microbial growth;

- technologies that remove or kill microorganisms in food.

These are useful distinctions but there are often areas of overlap.

Technologies that prevent contamination

Packaging

The living animal or plant which is used to make a food product has physical antimicrobial barriers such as the skin, shell, husk or rind to protect it from infection. These are often removed or damaged during processing to expose the underlying nutrient-rich material that can serve as an excellent medium for microbial growth. Packaging to some extent replaces these natural barriers. Traditional approaches are still common, such as the widespread use of banana leaves for packaging foods in tropical countries, the covering of cheeses in wax or immersing them in oil, and the wrapping of comminuted meat products in animal intestines. Modern technology has added numerous types of metal, glass, plastic and paper packaging to supplement these.

Generally the effect of packaging has been to improve food safety by protecting the food from contamination. Concern has been expressed about the migration of compounds present in packaging into some foods but, provided food-grade packaging materials are used, the levels of the compounds detected are minute and probably toxicologically insignificant. Lead soldered cans were once an important source of dietary lead but this has been controlled by the replacement of lead solder with electrically welded or two-piece cans.

Packaging sometimes also plays an important role in controlling the growth of microorganisms already present in the food when it is packed. In vacuum or modified atmosphere packaging, the packaging film is chosen for its gas permeability properties which determine whether it can retain an atmosphere inside the pack that is inhibitory to the growth of spoilage organisms. This can sometimes have safety implications since pathogens in general are little affected by this type of storage. Recognition of spoilage can be a warning of a potential safety risk since it signals that storage conditions have allowed extensive microbial growth to occur. If pathogens are unaffected by a packaging technology but spoilage is less obvious or delayed, there is an increased risk that unsafe foods will be consumed. This has led to outbreaks of botulism caused by vacuum-packed smoked fish in the past.

Cleaning and disinfection of equipment and utensils

The equipment used in food processing can act as a source of contamination if it is not thoroughly cleaned and disinfected. Cleaning has two objectives — removal of food residues adhering to the equipment which can support the growth of microorganisms, and removal of viable microorganisms. Both objectives can normally be achieved by washing in very hot water (around 80°C) or thorough washing with water and detergent followed by a sanitiser such as hypochlorite, iodophors or quaternary ammonium compounds to eliminate microorganisms that may still be adhering (Figure 5.1).

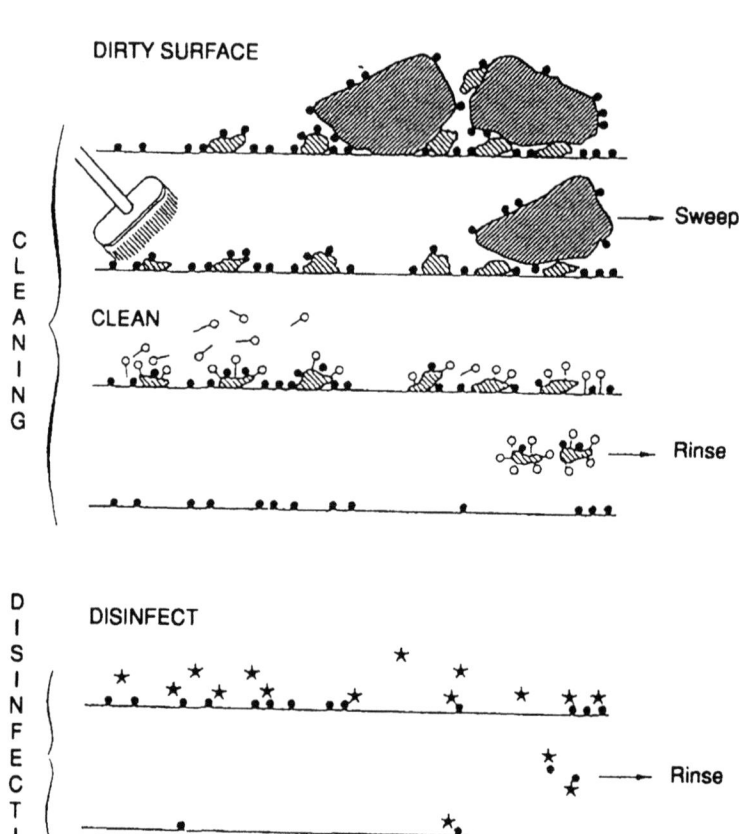

Figure 5.1 *Cleaning and disinfection*

Hygienic design of equipment

To ensure that equipment can be easily disinfected it must be designed and built with hygiene in mind. This will mean that it is free from pockets or crevices where food can accumulate and serve as a focus of infection, that it is easy to clean and disinfect, and that it is made from materials that will not contaminate the food and are unaffected by the cleaning and sanitizing agents used.

Technologies that control microbial growth

Chapter 3 described the factors that influence microbial growth. Many food preservation technologies, both traditional and modern, are based on the manipulation of one or several of these factors to inhibit microbial growth in food.

Decreasing the temperature can prevent or slow the growth of microorganisms depending on the temperature and the microorganisms concerned. Chill temperatures (< 8°) will prevent the growth of mesophilic bacterial pathogens such as *Salmonella, Shigella, E. coli* and *Clostridium perfringens* and psychrotrophs such as *Listeria monocytogenes* will grow only relatively slowly. Chilling does not necessarily eliminate a hazard though it can help control it. If the pathogen is present in high numbers before chilling, or if chill temperatures are not maintained throughout the storage period, a chilled food may still cause illness.

Microorganisms will not grow at temperatures below about -10°C. Frozen storage prevents their growth by the combined effect of the low temperature and the low water availability/activity (since much of the water will be ice). When foods are frozen some of the bacteria are killed or injured but many will survive and can resume growth if the food is defrosted and stored at a temperature within the danger zone. Helminths such as *Anisakis* and *Clonorchis* in fish and *Trichinella* and *Taenia* in meat are much more sensitive and can be killed by frozen storage at -20°C for seven days. In this context, freezing can be considered as a technology that eliminates a hazard. It is therefore of great potential importance in controlling foodborne helminth infections in countries where raw or lightly cooked fish and meats are eaten.

Many traditional food products rely on acidity to reduce the pH and inhibit the growth of pathogens and spoilage organisms. This acidity can be added in the form of vinegar (acetic acid) as in many traditional pickled products; lime or lemon juice (citric acid) as in some marinades and dressings; or it may be generated by lactic acid bacteria growing in the product to produce lactic acid as occurs in cheese, sauerkraut, yoghurt and salami production. At pH values where growth is prevented, microorganisms will eventually die though this can be quite a slow process, particularly at chill temperatures. It is therefore safest to regard acidification as a process which reduces risk rather than eliminates it.

Reducing the water availability/activity in a food by drying, salt-curing or conserving in sugar will also inhibit microbial growth. This is a widespread traditional food preservation technique. Microorganisms will generally survive this process even if they cannot grow in the final product. They could therefore resume growth if the product is rehydrated or stored in a moist environment where water will condense on the product increasing its a_w.

Modified atmosphere packaging and vacuum packaging of foods inhibit the growth of some microorganisms, principally those associated with spoilage, by increasing the level of carbon dioxide in the pack. Since maintenance of the appropriate gas atmosphere around the food depends on the packaging material, some of the safety implications of modified atmosphere packaging and vacuum packaging have already been discussed above.

Other antimicrobial agents such as nitrite, the bacteriocin nisin and benzoic acid are used in foods where their contribution is usually the inhibition of specific groups of organisms. Their effect is also often dependent on other environmental factors such as temperature and pH and illustrates an important concept in food preservation — the multiple barrier or hurdle concept. Changing a single factor that affects microbial growth in order to preserve a food often causes major changes in the food's characteristics and these are not always acceptable to the consumer. Acceptable shelf life and safety can often be achieved by adjusting a number of factors simultaneously. Each on its own is not sufficient to produce a useful inhibition of spoilage and/or pathogenic organisms but their cumulative effect is. Many traditional products are examples of the practical application of the hurdle concept. For example, the shelf life and safety of fermented meats such as salami depends on reductions in pH and water activity through drying and salting, the antimicrobial effect of nitrite and, in some cases, the preservative value of the chemicals deposited on the product as a result of smoking. Depending on the precise formulation, each of these can make a different contribution. Where the aggregate effect is insufficient, additional hurdles such as low temperature storage can also be employed. Similar multiple hurdles can be identified in cured meats, smoked fish, conserves and many other products.

Technologies that remove or kill microorganisms in food

Heat treatment

Various forms of cooking such as boiling, frying, roasting and baking have been used since earliest times to improve the palatability, digestibility and safety of foods. Even today, heat treatment remains the most accessible and effective method of ensuring that food is free from pathogenic organisms. Failure to deliver a sufficient heat process is often identified as a causative factor in outbreaks of foodborne illness.

The way in which we describe and measure how effectively a heat process kills microorganisms is described in Chapter 3. Heat treatments that kill only the vegetative forms of pathogens are called pasteurization. These can be applied to ensure the safety of liquid food products such as milk, liquid egg and ice cream mix, and the precise combination of time and temperature required to do this is normally prescribed in a regulation (see Table 4.2). Pasteurization is also used to extend the shelf life of products such as fruit juices, alcoholic and non-alcoholic drinks, pickles and sauces. The food safety risk from these products is usually very small due to other antimicrobial factors, particularly pH, though occasional outbreaks have been reported, such as an outbreak of *E. coli* O157 infection in the USA from contaminated apple juice.

Wherever it is applied, therefore, pasteurization provides an additional guarantee of safety.

Outbreaks of foodborne illness caused by pasteurized foods such as milk are generally the result of one of two possible failings:

- failure to apply a heat process sufficient to kill all vegetative pathogens present;
- contamination of the product after pasteurization from an unpasteurized product or from some other environmental source of pathogens.

Heat treatments more severe than pasteurization are also applied to foods. These kill all microorganisms capable of growth in the food under normal conditions of storage, including the more heat-resistant bacterial spores, resulting in shelf-stable products. These foods are described as being "commercially sterile" or appertized. Two techniques are used to produce appertized foods: canning and UHT processing coupled with aseptic packing.

Canned foods

All the food groups described in Chapter 4 can be processed into canned foods. These have an extremely good safety record and can normally be consumed, with or without reheating, with little fear of their causing illness. The product is packed into a container, normally a tin-plated can, sealed and then given a heat process far in excess of normal cooking which eliminates both the spores and the vegetative bacteria capable of causing spoilage or illness. This requires heating the product in the can to temperatures in excess of 100°C (normally around 121°C) for several minutes. It means that the product is stable for long periods without refrigeration.

Problems could arise if the product is insufficiently heated or if it is contaminated after heat processing. Commercially, the heat process is carefully designed, monitored and controlled to ensure that it achieves the desired reduction of bacterial spores. The principal food safety concern is that in low-acid foods (pH >4.5) the heat process must eliminate spores of *Clostridium botulinum*. A minimum heat process, known as a botulinum or 12D cook, is prescribed which reduces the number of *C. botulinum* spores by a factor of 10^{12} (1000 billion). In fact, to reduce the number of spores of spoilage organisms present to acceptably low levels, the heat process applied in practice is often far in excess of this safety minimum. Where the pH of the food is less than 4.5, *Clostridium botulinum* will not grow even if the spores survive and so a milder heat process can be used. Safety problems can arise when low acid (pH >4.5) foods are canned or bottled at home where the potential safety problems are less well understood and control is less stringent. A number of outbreaks of botulism have been associated with home-bottled vegetables in the past.

When the hot cans are cooled after processing, a vacuum is created inside the can which could result in contamination being sucked in from outside. An outbreak of typhoid fever was caused in just this way when cans of corned beef were cooled in contaminated river water. To prevent this from happening, clean chlorinated water should always be used for cooling.

Cans are protected from recontamination by the strength and integrity of the container. A key part of this is the complex double seam which joins the can lid to its base (Figure 5.2). Checking the

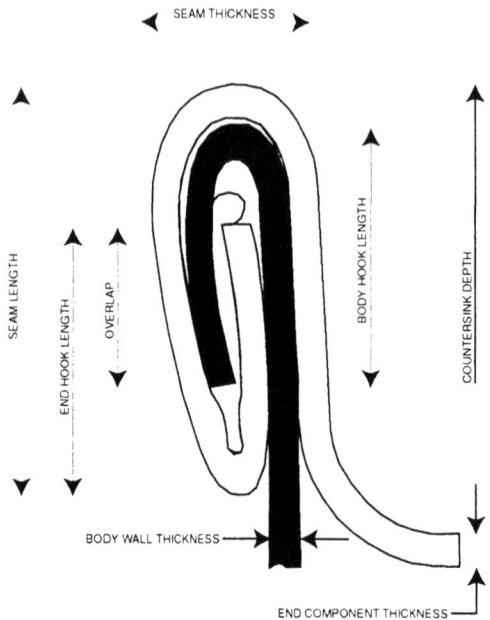

Figure 5.2 *The double seam can*

seam to ensure that it is correctly formed is an important safety control measure. To do this thoroughly requires some expertise but gross failures are more readily detected (Figure 5.3).

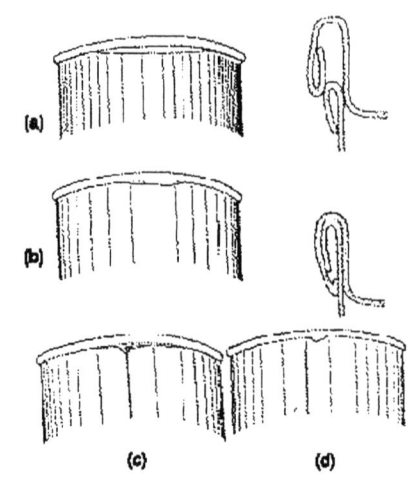

Figure 5.3 *Defects in can seams*

Physical damage or deterioration of the can could also lead to contamination of its contents. Often microbial growth in a can will become apparent when gas is produced and the end of the can swells. Food from cans which have deformed in this way should not be eaten. However, this may not always happen so food must also be discarded when it comes from cans that are dented or rusty or where the food appears "off" once the can is opened.

If they are not used immediately on opening, the contents of a can should be transferred to a clean dry container for storage. Food should never be left in an open can as this can lead to increased uptake of tin from the container.

UHT processing/aseptic packaging

In these processes the food is heat-treated before being packaged in a previously sterilized container in a sterile environment. By heating the product separately its temperature can be increased much more quickly, often to temperatures higher than those used in canning, and this reduces quality losses in the product while retaining the same antimicrobial effect. The packaging material is usually a plastic or laminate film that is formed into containers in the packaging machine, though sometimes preformed containers are also used. In most commercial equipment the packaging is sterilized by hot hydrogen peroxide.

UHT processing is applied mainly to liquid foods such as milk, soups and fruit juices because they heat up very quickly as a result of convection. If a food contains particles that heat up by conduction, the process is slower and some of the advantages of UHT processing are lost. New techniques such as ohmic heating which will heat particulates rapidly promise an extension of UHT processing to other foods.

Ionizing irradiation

Specific applications of radiation treatments are now permitted in more than 35 countries. These include the treatment of meat, poultry, eggs and shrimps to remove parasites and *Salmonella* and the decontamination of food ingredients such as spices and herbs. Parasites are more sensitive to irradiation than bacteria and doses as low as 0.3 kGy can render them non-infective. Bacterial spores are relatively resistant (Table 5.1).

At the low doses allowed to remove vegetative forms of bacteria (<10 kGy), no perceptible changes are produced in the food so it retains the characteristics of the raw product.

Concerns over the potential safety of food irradiation have been extensively investigated and found to be without foundation. Despite its undoubted potential to contribute to food safety, commercial uptake of irradiation has been limited because of consumer resistance to the concept of irradiated foods.

Ultraviolet irradiation

Ultraviolet light can kill microorganisms but, unlike ionizing radiation, its penetrating power is very limited. Its use is restricted to disinfecting surfaces and also reducing the population of airborne fungal spores in areas where they would pose a threat to a product's shelf life (e.g. in bakeries).

Washing and disinfection

Washing with clean water will remove some of the microorganisms adhering to the surface of a food product. The numbers of microorganisms on the food can be reduced still further if the water used contains an antimicrobial compound such as chlorine which will kill some of those that remain attached to the surface. Washing fruits and vegetables is an obvious example of this. While it is a useful and effective safety measure for reducing gross contamination, microorganisms in surface pockets inaccessible to the water and antimicrobial will be unaffected.

Table 5.1 *Dose requirement in various applications of food irradiation*

Purpose	Dose (kGy)	Products
Low dose (up to 1 kGy)		
Inhibition of sprouting	0.05-0.15	Potatoes, onions, garlic, gingerroot, etc.
Insect disinfestation and parasite disinfection	0.15-0.50	Cereals and pulses, fresh and dried fruits, dried fish and meat, fresh pork, etc
Delay of physiological process (e.g. ripening)	0.5-1.0	Fresh fruits and vegetables
Medium dose (1-10 kGy)		
Extension of shelf-life	1.0-3.0	Fresh fish, strawberries, etc.
Elimination of spoilage and pathogenic microorganisms	1.0-7.0	Fresh and frozen seafood, raw or frozen poultry and meat, etc.
Improving technological properties of food	2.0-7.0	Grapes (increasing juice yield), dehydrated vegetables /reduced cooking time), etc.
High dose (10-50 kGy)		
Industrial sterilization (in combination with mild heat)	30-50	Meat, poultry, seafood, prepared foods, sterilized hospital diets
Decontamination of certain additives and ingredients	10-50	Spices, enzyme preparations, natural gums, etc.

Washing meat carcasses with solutions of organic acids such as lactic acid has been used in some countries as a means of reducing surface contamination.

Leaving foods wet after washing can actually encourage microbial growth as the availability of water will be increased for those microorganisms that have survived the treatment.

Water itself can be disinfected by boiling or by the addition of chlorine or a chlorine-based sanitizer to a point where there is residual free chlorine detectable in the water. Some pathogenic protozoa such as *Cryptosporidium* show a marked resistance to chlorine and can be effectively removed from water only by filtration. Therefore to produce a safe water combination of filtration and disinfection is recommended.

KEY POINTS

- Food preservation technologies can be classified according to their effect on microorganisms.

- Some technologies prevent contamination.

- Some technologies control microbial growth and production of toxin.

- Some technologies remove or kill microorganisms in food.

- If correctly applied, these technologies improve the keeping quality and safety of food.

- Processes that kill microorganisms give the greatest certainty of food safety.

- Heat treatment is the most effective and accessible method of killing microorganisms in foods.

Chapter 6
Hygiene in food preparation

Chapter 3 describes the principal sources of food contamination and these are mentioned again in the discussion of the safety of particular food commodities in Chapter 4. Clearly it is important to be aware of specific problems associated with certain foods. However, in many cases, food safety can be enhanced by a number of general measures, regardless of the food materials being handled. The most important of these have been formulated by WHO as a set of *Ten golden rules for safe food preparation*. These are presented in Appendix 2. These give guidance to the general population on the essential principles of safe food preparation.

Though the *Ten golden rules* apply equally to all food preparation activities, catering on a larger scale is a more complex operation than preparing food for the immediate family and requires more detailed rules. It involves preparing larger quantities of food for more people mainly using paid employees, special premises and equipment. It is also becoming increasingly important as more people eat food that has been prepared outside the home, at work, in hospitals and educational establishments, at social gatherings and so on. The scale of mass catering means that breakdowns in good hygienic practices can have far more serious consequences in terms of the number of people affected and, sadly, events involving mass catering often feature prominently in many national statistics on outbreaks of foodborne illness. For these reasons a more extended list of food hygiene requirements directed at mass catering is given here. The reader is also referred to other WHO publications dealing specifically with this topic. (See bibliography) Many of the rules apply to food preparation at all levels, though some are excessive and inappropriate to food preparation in the home. Some instances of this are highlighted.

Rules of good hygienic practices in food preparation deal broadly with three different areas: physical factors relating to the premises and equipment used, operational factors relating to the hygienic handling of food, and personal factors relating to questions of personal hygiene and training (Figure 6.1).

Physical Factors

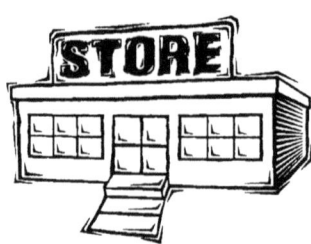

Buildings, location, layout, equipment

Processing Factors

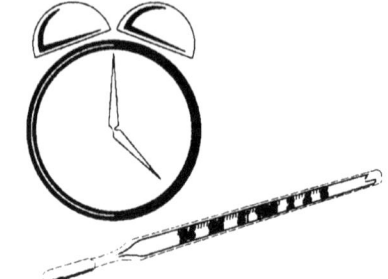

Time/temperature contamination

Personal Factors

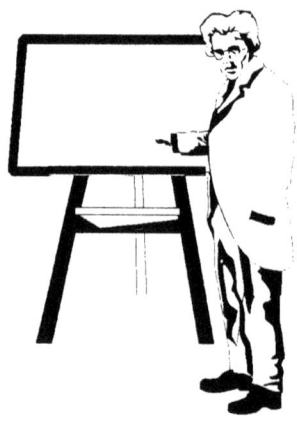

Training

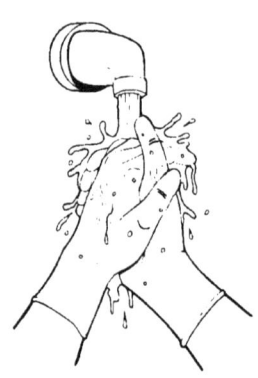

Personal hygiene

Figure 6.1 *Principle components of food hygiene*

Physical factors: premises and equipment

Ideally, food preparation premises should be purpose built and sited in an area that is free from objectionable odours, smoke and dust, is located away from rubbish tips, and is not prone to events such as flooding. In practice one usually has a more limited choice about the building to be used and its location, but it should be of sound construction and well maintained.

A first requirement is that the working environment should be well lit, well ventilated and tidy as this will encourage good working practices and promote food safety. The working environment should also be clean and easy to clean. Microorganisms can grow on any scrap or particle of food remaining on food contact surfaces or lodged in some crack or crevice and this can act as a source of contamination. While most microorganisms will be associated with food particles that can be removed by thorough physical cleaning, it should be remembered that a surface may appear physically clean although it may not be microbiologically clean. In commercial food processing this is overcome by using an antimicrobial agent (a disinfectant or sanitizer) as well as a detergent to clean food contact surfaces. This can be expensive and unnecessary at the household level. Heat is the most effective antimicrobial agent and thorough washing with hot water (more than 80°C), perhaps with a small amount of detergent, will clean a surface and kill those microorganisms that are not easily removed (Figure 5.1). Frequent cleaning is also important since dried and encrusted residues are much harder to remove.

Cloths used for cleaning can rapidly accumulate a large population of microorganisms, particularly when left moist, and their use can actually increase contamination rather than reduce it. They should therefore be changed every day and boiled before re-use.

We have already seen how raw foods can act as a source of pathogens. It is important, therefore, that the layout of the premises and equipment should allow foods to be stored and handled without contact between raw and cooked products, either directly or via equipment.

The food should also be protected from other sources of contamination such as soil, insects, rodents and other animals (wild or domesticated). For this reason, food should not be placed on or near the ground in open containers. As far as possible, the premises should be protected to prevent pests entering. This is sometimes very difficult in the household so storing foods in tightly sealed containers is an effective second line of defence.

Facilities should also be available for storing dangerous or toxic substances such as disinfectants and insecticides outside the kitchen area in a clearly marked location. This will minimize the risk of accidents occurring as a result of confusion between poisonous substances and food materials. Rubbish and waste should also be stored away from the food preparation area.

The importance of not leaving food for extended periods at temperatures in the danger zone at which microbial growth can occur has been referred to earlier. The equipment used to cool food is of obvious importance here. For example, shallow trays allow faster cooling of foods and are preferable to deeper containers. Cold storage equipment should be well maintained and checked regularly to ensure it operates at the correct temperature. If cold storage equipment is overloaded this will slow down the cooling process and the food will spend longer in the temperature danger zone.

Similarly, cooking equipment should be adequate for its intended use, well maintained and checked regularly to confirm that it is functioning correctly.

To allow good personal hygiene, the premises must have adequate and hygienic toilet facilities separated from the food production area, as well as adequate hand-washing facilities.

Operational factors: hygienic handling of food

A large part of the hygienic handling of foods relates to the correct use of temperature in the control of microorganisms — avoiding temperatures where microbial growth is possible and, where appropriate, ensuring that temperatures are sufficiently high to kill microorganisms. For example, perishable foods should normally be stored refrigerated at <10°C. Food that are cooked should be cooked thoroughly to ensure that all parts reach a temperature of at least 70°C. Precooked foods should be stored outside the temperature danger zone of 10–60°C and those served hot should be reheated to 70°C before consumption.

If frozen meat and poultry are not completely defrosted before cooking, some parts may not get hot enough to kill the pathogens present.

When dishes containing a mixture of cooked and raw ingredients are being prepared, it is important to cool the cooked component before mixing with the other ingredients. Failure to do this could lead to a temporary rise in temperature during which microbial growth can occur.

The other major objective of hygienic food handling is to avoid contamination, particularly of cooked or ready-to-eat foods. Physical measures such as the exclusion of vermin from the premises contribute to this, as do a number of operational procedures such as keeping food covered as much as possible.

The liquid that accumulates during the defrosting of frozen meat is likely to contain pathogenic microorganisms. It must not be allowed to drip on other foods stored below it and great care must be taken in disposing of it. Any equipment or surfaces contaminated during defrosting must be thoroughly cleaned and disinfected.

Cooked food should be kept well separated from raw food to reduce the risk of cross-contamination.

Touching cooked foods with bare hands should be avoided wherever possible as even clean hands can carry pathogenic microorganisms. Ideally, hair should be covered or at the very least tied back when one is working in a kitchen. Hair in food is not just aesthetically objectionable but may also be a source of pathogens.

Personal factors: personal hygiene and training

As indicated in Chapter 3, the food handler can often be a major source of contamination. There are several good hygienic practices that he or she should observe.

Hands should be washed regularly with soap in clean water, but especially before starting to handle food, after going to the toilet or changing a baby, and after handling raw food, food waste or chemicals. In all these activities the hands may become contaminated with pathogens or toxic chemical residues that can then be transferred to the food. It is easier to keep hands clean if finger nails are kept short and jewellery such as rings are removed as dirt can become lodged under these and may be difficult to remove.

Food handlers should avoid coughing into their hands or touching their hair, nose or mouth while handling food without washing their hands afterwards.

Routine medical and microbiological examination of food handlers is not generally recommended but if food handlers are suffering from an illness that includes symptoms such as jaundice, diarrhoea, vomiting, fever, sore throat, skin rash or skin lesions such as boils or cuts, they should report this to their supervisor before starting work. It may then be necessary for them to be assigned temporarily to some other task which does not involve handling food. This should not leave the worker financially worse off as it would then be a disincentive to the honest disclosure of any symptoms.

A person suffering from diarrhoea should not be allowed to handle open food. If food is to be handled by a person with spots or infected cuts or skin lesions, these should be covered with a waterproof dressing.

It is not necessary for a food handler to have an overt infection in order to pose a threat to food safety. The asymptomatic carriage of *Staphylococcus aureus* on the skin, in the nasopharynx and hair follicles has already been described. Activities that encourage hand/mouth contact such as smoking or the chewing of gum, tobacco, betel nut or finger nails can also therefore lead to food contamination and must be avoided. The same also applies to the tasting of food during preparation. Similarly, food handlers should not spit, sneeze or cough over food, or pick their nose, ears or any other parts of their body.

Many of the basic rules of food hygiene are already observed as part of traditional religious or cultural habits that go back thousands of years, but the reasons for their importance in terms of food safety are often not clearly understood. It is easy for lapses to occur resulting in a threat to food safety. Education of food handlers in basic food hygiene is important so that rules are not seen as pointless irritants dreamed up by bureaucrats. If food handlers understand the reasons for the rules, this will encourage them to apply the rules rigorously and consistently. For the general population, basic food hygiene education can focus on WHO's *Ten golden rules* but more detailed training is required for food handlers in mass catering. In this educational process, the health worker can play a significant role. This is one of the issues addressed in Chapter 7.

The Hazard Analysis and Critical Control Point (HACCP) system

Where general rules of good food hygiene are followed, they establish a baseline of good practice in food preparation that can play an important role in ensuring food safety. The strength of such rules lies in their general applicability, but this can also be a source of weakness. In attempting to cover all circumstances, some rules may seem vague, or even irrelevant or unrealistic in certain situations, and to some this can appear to devalue the whole approach. Individual food preparation activities, both domestic and on a larger scale, have their own characteristics: they do not all produce the same products, and they use different raw materials, different processes and different equipment. What food handlers really want is guidance on food safety related to their own specific operations. Precisely how should they store their raw materials? What are the most important areas to clean and when (sweeping a dusty floor, for instance, is cleaning but it can actually increase contamination of exposed food)? How long should the food be cooked? In what order should ingredients be added? These and many other questions are often of great relevance to food safety and require specific answers.

One approach to checking the safety of particular foods would be to test them to see if they contain specific pathogens or other organisms that might indicate the presence of pathogens. This is a totally unrealistic option for domestic and small-scale food preparation and, while at first sight appealing, it has been discredited even for large-scale food production. It is now almost universally recognized that microbiological testing of food products on its own is an ineffective and expensive way of trying to achieve an acceptable level of food safety assurance.

Microbiological testing can be very costly and only gives information after the event, when the problem has already arisen. It may also give a false sense of security since microorganisms will not be spread uniformly throughout a food and samples taken may not show the presence of pathogens even though the food is contaminated. Even when pathogens are detected, this will not necessarily indicate where the problem arose and how it can be solved. Without this information, the same problem is likely to recur again and again.

A far better approach is to control microbiological quality at source, during production or preparation, so that safety is built into the product. Put simply, it is much better to prevent a problem from arising than try to remedy the situation after it has. Food hygiene rules attempt to do this but lack the specificity required. To overcome this problem, new preventative approaches have had to be developed. The most commonly implemented of these is known as the system of Hazard Analysis and Critical Control Point (HACCP).

HACCP involves the systematic evaluation of a specific food processing or preparation procedure to identify hazards associated with ingredients or the processing procedure itself and to find out how those hazards can be controlled. It then decides which steps in the process are essential to controlling hazards so that attention can be focused on them.

While this system was first applied to commercial food processing, it can also be applied to any operation where food is handled or processed for consumption. It is also replacing traditional regulatory approaches. Many countries now recognize HACCP in their food safety regulations and their enforcement procedures are being adapted to ensure that food industries apply HACCP in a systematic way.

The full rigours of a HACCP system, as outlined in Appendix 3, are probably not feasible or even necessary in households, but the essence of the approach — identifying hazards and the key steps that will ensure their control is useful both at the level of the household and more generally in health education campaigns and courses.

KEY POINTS

- Application of general rules governing food hygiene can improve food safety.

- WHO's *Ten Golden Rules for Safe Food Preparation* summarize the most important aspects of food hygiene.

- More detailed rules are required for mass catering than for domestic food preparation.

- Hygiene rules govern physical, operational and personal factors.

- Health workers can play an important role in educating food handlers in food hygiene.

- General rules suffer from a lack of specificity.

- Microbiological testing of food, while specific, is ineffective as a routine tool for assuring food safety.

- Application of procedures that are both preventive and specific such as HACCP are the most effective way of protecting food safety.

Chapter 7
The role of health workers in food safety

The first six chapters describe the basics of foodborne illness: what it is, the factors that lead to it, the problems associated with specific foods and food processing, and how these factors might be controlled. We now consider what the health worker can do to alleviate the problem of foodborne illness, particularly with regard to children.

The health worker has essentially three roles: curative, preventive and surveillance.

The curative role

In many cases the immediate problem faced by the health worker is how to deal with a sick patient. The foodborne origin of an illness may not be immediately apparent for, although many foodborne illnesses have diarrhoea as a principal symptom, others can have a variety of presentations. It is not the intention of this book to provide a manual on the treatment of foodborne illness. Much of this should already be a key part of a health worker's training and there are a number of other publications that deal specifically with this aspect (see bibliography).

Reliance on treatment, however successful, has its limitations. Treatment of an infected individual does not remove the cause of illness from the environment or eliminate behaviours that lead to foodborne illness. It does not, therefore, prevent other people from becoming ill by the same route. Nor does infection necessarily confer protection and reduce the risk of a patient succumbing to another episode soon after recovery. So while treatment remains an essential task for the health worker, recognition of its limitations has led to greater emphasis being placed on preventive measures to reduce the overall incidence of illness.

The preventive role: controlling foodborne hazards

The health worker can intervene to reduce the incidence of foodborne illness through food safety education programmes. Cases of diarrhoeal disease, for instance, should prompt the health worker to consider whether food is being prepared correctly. The mother or other care-giver who brings a child for treatment can be given information about how to avoid foodborne hazards by correct food preparation. A group of cases of diarrhoeal disease would be an opportunity to give educational messages to the whole community. In this way the health worker plays not only a reactive (curative) role but also a proactive (preventive) one. The situation varies from country to country and it is not possible to prescribe one approach to prevention that will work equally well everywhere. However, some suggestions are given here that may be adapted to different situations.

Food safety education programmes should aim to improve the knowledge and practice of an entire population (including policy-makers, food producers, food processors, professional food handlers and consumers), as all have a role to play in food safety. However, certain groups, either because of their direct role in food preparation and/or increased vulnerability to foodborne diseases need to receive greater emphasis in the programme. These groups are:

- *domestic food handlers* who prepare food for the family, particularly expectant mothers and mothers with small children who are especially vulnerable;

- *professional food handlers* such as street food vendors, catering personnel and those working in the food processing industry (in feeding large numbers of people their impact on overall food safety is considerable);

- *high-risk groups and people preparing food for them*, particularly small children, travellers, pregnant women, the immunocompromised and the elderly.

Domestic food handlers

Domestic food handlers are persons who prepare food for consumption by their families. Experience has shown that a large proportion of foodborne disease outbreaks occur in the home as a result of mishandling of food. Education of this target group will help domestic food handlers to protect themselves and their family members. Particular attention should be given to WHO's *Ten Golden Rules for Safe Food Preparation* (Appendix 2).

Expectant mothers

There are a number of foodborne infections, notably listeriosis and toxoplasmosis, which may adversely affect the foetus. Chemical contaminants such as lead or methyl mercury, depending on their level of intake, may also have negative effect on the health of the foetus. Pregnant women are often motivated to do all they can for the health of their baby. Health workers — particularly those in maternal and child health centres and primary health care centres — have the responsibility of informing women on the type of food/practices which may present greater risks. Education of expectant mothers in food safety should include information on breast-feeding. A WHO brochure providing advice on food safety issues of importance to pregnant women is also under preparation.

Lactating women

Breast milk is the ideal source of nourishment and the safest food for infants during the first 4–6 months of life. It protects them against foodborne diarrhoea through its anti-infective properties and by minimizing exposure to foodborne pathogens. Major efforts are being made at national and international levels to promote breast-feeding, and a great deal of educational material is available for advising mothers on this subject. Health workers can also advise lactating women how to protect their breast milk from chemical or other hazards (e.g. by minimizing contact with pesticides, by avoiding consumption of foods containing unsafe levels of contaminants).

Mothers of older infants and young children

While public health authorities have recognized the importance of breast-feeding in preventing foodborne diseases, almost no attention has been paid to safe food handling during the preparation of complementary foods. The education of mothers and care-givers in food safety principles is vital if there is to be a substantial improvement in prevention of diarrhoeal diseases in infants and children. In this area, health workers clearly have the leading role. Most health centres already advise mothers on breast-feeding, infant feeding and nutrition, as well as other aspects of the care of infants and children. It would be important that these centres extend their information and education to include information on safe food handling practices. WHO has issued a leaflet entitled *Basic principles for preparation of safe food for infants and young children* that health workers can use for advising mothers in food safety.

Professional food handlers

Professional food handlers should ideally receive training and education in two aspects of food safety:

a) *principles of good hygienic practice*;

b) *application of the HACCP concept to food preparation*.

Where food handlers are receiving formal training and education in food preparation, the above two aspects of food safety should be included in their curricula. Training in principles of good hygienic practice equip food handlers with the rudiments of food safety whereas training in HACCP helps them to learn to adopt a critical thought process and eventually learn to:

- identify potential hazards and control measures that are relevant, effective and specific to the operation in question and to the work situation;

- prioritize control measures, ensure that the critical ones are applied correctly and that they meet the necessary conditions; and

- to take appropriate action when conditions are not met.

When food handlers lack professional training and qualifications, its may be difficult to train them in HACCP. In such cases, it is nevertheless important to impress on them the value of this technique. Health authorities or health workers could assist in conducting HACCP studies by identifying hazards, appropriate control measures, critical control points, critical limits and corrective measures and train food handlers in the outcome of the studies.

High-risk groups and people preparing food for them

Travellers

Travellers will require advice on safe and unsafe foods in a particular area. If a region has a reputation for unsafe food, income from tourism could be affected. Travellers often consult physicians or clinics for vaccination and other prophylactic or therapeutic treatment. Advice on prevailing foodborne diseases and on food and drink likely to be contaminated in certain countries could be provided to travellers at vaccination centres. WHO has issued a guide on safe food for travellers that is intended to help meet this need (see bibliography).

The elderly

The elderly constitute an increasing proportion of the population. They must be made aware that the health consequences of foodborne infections may be more serious for them, and that they may be more susceptible than other groups to infections such as salmonellosis, enterohaemorrhagic *E. coli* infection and listeriosis. Health workers in contact with the elderly can encourage them to avoid high-risk foods such as meals made from raw or undercooked animal products (eggs, meat, milk) or raw seafood.

The sick

Great care should be taken when preparing food for hospital patients — including the newborn if they are not breastfed. Food handlers in hospital kitchens should be trained in safe food handling. Nurses and dieticians should also receive education in food safety. The highest standards of hygiene will be required for foods produced for the sick and elderly.

It should be remembered that the standard of cleanliness and hygienic practice in health centres sets an example for visitors. A poor standard of hygiene in these places will have a negative effect while good hygienic practices will encourage visitors to emulate them.

The undernourished

Undernourished persons are especially susceptible to foodborne diseases and should therefore also be seen as an important target group for educational interventions.

The community

The whole community should participate in health education in food safety. In their dealings with members of high-risk target groups and with the community members in general, health workers should ensure that all understand the *Ten Golden Rules for Safe Food Preparation* recommended by WHO.

Refugees

When disaster strikes, the safety of the food supply may be affected, leading to a greater risk of foodborne disease. At the same time, people may flee their homes and the situation of refugees and displaced persons requires special care and attention. Conditions in refugee camps are prone to outbreaks of foodborne disease. Environmental contamination and improper food handling increase the risk of epidemics such as cholera. While education of the public in food safety is important at all times, in disasters and emergencies it is an absolute necessity. When there is a risk of epidemics, families should be reminded of the rules of safe food handling.

Mass feeding in refugee camps has many advantages. It ensures, for instance that food is available to everyone. However, there are also disadvantages in that it increases the risk of large scale outbreaks of foodborne illness. In refugee centres, food handlers who are responsible for preparing the food, and their supervisors, need training in safe food handling and in the HACCP concept. Health workers can give them clear instructions about their responsibilities and may even put up posters with the rules for safe food handling. Health workers should make sure that those responsible for the refugee centre understand the important need for adequate clean water and sanitation, and for proper disposal of unused food and other waste.

Schoolchildren

Schoolchildren are both a target group for education on food safety and a channel for this education as well. Educating school children is a very effective strategy for preventing foodborne diseases as the children not only learn about food safety themselves but also communicate the need for food hygiene to their parents and other family members. The earlier that education in food safety starts, the better it is. Even children in kindergartens and nurseries can be trained in some basic rules of food hygiene. Teaching children about food safety has the doubly beneficial effect of helping to protect a vulnerable group and of educating the next generation.

In many places, existing school education on food safety is limited to teaching about hand-washing after defecation, protection from flies and rodents, latrine use and safe storage of water. Although this advice is important, it has not always been enough to prevent foodborne illness, which more often results from insufficient cooking, incorrect storage of food, re-use of leftovers, lack of hand-washing prior to food preparation, and other factors that favour contamination, survival and multiplication of pathogens, or production of toxins in food.

Teachers may themselves have no education in the subject, and may often lack teaching materials. Therefore, if teaching about food safety is to be improved, teachers should also receive formal training in food safety. Where food safety is not on the school curriculum, this presents an opportunity for health workers to visit schools to educate children about the importance of food hygiene.

Street food vendors and food service establishments

A substantial amount of food handling and processing occurs in street food vending operations and food service establishments. In many situations it is not possible to control these operations completely through official inspection. Control must be exercised by the food handlers themselves. The role of the health worker in helping this to happen is to provide both the food handlers and the consumers with information and education about food safety.

Surveillance

Health workers should actively participate in the surveillance of foodborne diseases. Epidemiological data are needed so that public health authorities can be aware of the kind of diseases that are current in the population, can identify which population subgroups are most at risk, can plan appropriate food safety programmes, and can target educational interventions in an appropriate way. Surveillance of diseases involves five methods:

- registration of deaths and hospital discharge diagnoses;
- disease notification;
- sentinel surveillance;
- laboratory surveillance;
- outbreak investigation.

In most countries, physicians complete a death certificate when a person in their care dies. In many hospitals, and in all hospitals in some countries, hospital records include data on the diagnosis of all patients who are discharged.

Notification of diseases is often legally required from physicians or other health workers, though this notification may apply only to certain conditions. This information is usually analysed centrally in order to identify trends in health and illness and also to detect outbreaks of disease.

In sentinel surveillance, selected health workers or facilities monitor selected health events. For foodborne diseases, relevant health events might include syndromes such as diarrhoea, dehydration and haemolytic uraemic syndrome, or specific infections such as campylobacteriosis, salmonellosis, or *E. coli* O157:H7 infection. Laboratory surveillance involves the recording of results of laboratory investigation of specimens (usually faecal samples) obtained from patients. The laboratory can test for a range of pathogens.

Outbreak detection takes several forms. Health workers should keep alert to the possibility of a shared exposure among patients with the same condition, or they may routinely report selected conditions either voluntarily or as required by law.

KEY POINTS

- Prevention is better than cure.

- Education in food safety is an important preventive measure.

- Educational programmes must be focused and relevant to the target audience.

- Specific target groups for food safety education should be identified and educational interventions aimed at them.

- Mothers and pregnant women are important target groups for prevention of infant diarrhoea.

- In addition to education of food handlers in basic principles of food hygiene, an HACCP-based approach can be applied to the preparation of food in homes, in food service establishments or for street food vending operations in order to select behaviours which are of particular importance to food safety.

- Surveillance of foodborne diseases is an important tool for assessing the food safety situation and identifying factors leading to foodborne diseases.

References

1. Kilbourne EM. et al. Toxic oil syndrome: a current clinical and epidemiological summary, including comparisons with the eosinophilia-myalgia syndrome. *J. Am. Coll. Cardiol.*, 1991, **18**:711–717.

2. Hall RL. *The flavour industry.* August 1971, p.455

3. Archer D, Young FE. Contemporary issues:diseases with a food vector. *Clinical Microbiology Reviews*, 1988, **1**:377–398.

4. Motarjemi Y. et al. Contaminated weaning food a major risk factor for diarrhoea and associated malnutrition. *Bulletin of the WHO*, 1993, **71**: 79–92.

5. ICMSF. Parasites. In: *Micro-organisms in foods, Vol. 5. Microbiological specifications of food pathogens.* London, Blackie, 1996, pp. 193–197.

6. Dim LA. et al. Lead and other metals distributed in local cooking salt from the Fofi salt spring in Akwana, Nigeria. *J. Environ. Sci. Health*, 1991, **B26**:357–365.

7. Jacopsen JL, Jacopsen SW. Intellectual impairment in children exposed to polychlorinated biphenyls in utero. *The New England journal of medicine*, 1996, **335**: 783–789.

8. Ferrer A, Cabral R. Toxic epidemics caused by alimentary exposure to pesticides: a review. *Food additives and contaminants*, 1991, **8**:755–776.

9. Centers for Disease Control. Lead-contaminated drinking water in bulk-water storage tanks — Arizona and California, 1993. *Morbidity and mortality weekly report*, 1994, **43**:751, 757–758.

10. Coultate TP. *Food: the chemistry of its components.* Cambridge, Royal Society of Chemistry, 1984, pp. 266–269.

11. Tylleskär TM et al. Cassava cyanogens and konzo, an upper motorneurone disease found in Africa. *Lancet*, **339**:208–211.

12. Nugon-Baudon L, Rabot S. Glucosinolates and glucosinolate derivatives: implications for protection against chemical carcinogenesis. *Nutrition research reviews*, 1994, **7**: 205–231.

13. Moss MO. Mycotoxins. *Mycological research*, 1996, **100**:513–523.

14. Smith JE, Solomons GL, Lewis CW, Anderson JG. *Mycotoxins in human nutrition and health.* European Commission CG XII, 1994.

15. Al Bustan MA, Udo EE, Chugh TD. Nasal carriage of enterotoxin producing *Staphylococcus aureus* among restaurant workers in Kuwait City. *Epidemiol. Infect.*, 1996, **116**:319–322.

16. St Louis ME, Peck SHS, Bowering D et al. *Annals of internal medicine*, 1988, **108**:363–368.

17. Lorri W, Svandberg U. Lower prevalence of diarrhoea in young children fed lactic acid fermented cereal gruels. *Food nutrition bulletin*, 1994, **15**:52–63.

18. Blake PA et al. Cholera in Portugal, 1974. *American journal of epidemiology*, 1997, **105**:337–348.

19. Fukjikawa, H. et al. Contamination of microbial foreign bodies in bottled mineral water in Tokyo, Japan. *J. Applied Microbiology*, 1997, **82**:287–291.

Bibliography

The WHO Ten golden rules for safe food preparation. Geneva, World Health Organization, 1989.

Hygiene in food-service and mass catering establishments. Important rules. Geneva, World Health Organization, 1994 (WHO document WHO/FNU/FOS/94.5).

Food safety measures for eggs & foods containing eggs. Geneva, World Health Organization, 1996 (WHO document WHO/FNU/FOS/96.5).

Basic principles for the preparation of safe food for infants and young children. Geneva, World Health Organization, 1996 (WHO document WHO/FNU/FOS/96.6).

Jacob M. *Safe food handling. A training guide for managers of food service establishments*. Geneva, World Health Organization, 1989.

Bryan FL. *Hazard analysis critical control point evaluations. A guide to identifying hazards and assessing risks associated with food preparation and storage*. Geneva, World Health Organization, 1992.

A guide on safe food for travellers. A leaflet that can help travellers avoid illness caused by unsafe food and drink. Geneva, World Health Organiztion, 1994.

Street-vended food: A HACCP-based food safety strategy for governments. Geneva, World Health Organization, 1995 (WHO document WHO/FNU/FOS/95.5)

Food safety. Examples of health education materials. Geneva, World Health Organization, 1989 (WHO document WHO/EHE/FOS/89.2).

The contamination of food. Nairobi, United Nations Environment Programme, 1992. (UNEP/GEMS Environmental Library, No. 5).

Williams T, Moon A, Williams M. *Food, environment and health. A guide for primary school teachers*. Geneva, World Health Organization, 1990.

Health surveillance and management procedures for food-handling personnel. Report of a WHO Consultation. Geneva, World Health Organization, 1989 (WHO Technical Report Series, No. 785).

Guidelines for cholera control. Geneva, World Health Organization, 1993.

Food technologies and public health. Geneva, World Health Organization, 1995 (WHO document WHO/FNU/FOS/95.12).

Fermentation: assessment and research. Report of a FAO/WHO Workshop. Geneva, World Health Organization, 1995 (WHO document WHO/FNU/FOS/95.11).

Food irradiation. A technique for preserving and improving the safety of food. Geneva, World Health Organization, 1988.

Training workshop on HACCP. Geneva, World Health Organization, 1996 (WHO document WHO/FNU/FOS/96.3).

Bibliography

International directory of audiovisual material on food safety. Geneva, World Health Organization, 1995 (WHO document WHO/FNU/FOS/95.4).

The role of food safety in health and development. Report of a Joint FAO/WHO Expert Committee on Food Safety, 1984. Geneva, World Health Organization, 1984 (WHO Technical Report Series, No. 705).

Evaluation of programmes to ensure food safety - guiding principles. Geneva, World Health Organization, 1989.

International Conference on Nutrition. *A challenge to the food safety community.* Geneva, World Health Organization, 1996 (WHO document WHO/FNU/FOS/96.4).

Guidelines for strengthening a national food safety programme. Geneva, World Health Organization, 1996 (WHO document WHO/FNU/96.2).

WHO surveillance programme for control of foodborne infections and intoxications in Europe. Sixth Report (1990-1992). Geneva, World Health Organization, 1992.

Borgdorff MW, Motarjemi Y. *Surveillance of foodborne diseases: what are the options?* Geneva, World Health Organization, 1997 (WHO document WHO/FSF/FOS/97.3).

The Treatment of Diarrhoea - A manual for physicians and other senior health workers. Geneva, World Health Organization, 1995 (WHO document WHO/CDR/95).

Advising mothers on management of diarrhoea in the home. Geneva, World Health Organization, 1993 (WHO document WHO/CDD/93.2)

The selection of fluids and food for home therapy to prevent dehydration from diarrhoea. Geneva, World Health Organization, 1995 (WHO document WHO/CDD/93.44)

A healthy pregnancy through a healthy diet. Geneva, World Health Organization (in preparation).

GEMS/FOOD International dietary survey: Infant Exposure to Certain Organochlorine Contaminants from Breast-Milk: a risk assessment. Geneva, World Health Organization, 1998 (WHO document WHO/FSF/FOS/98.4).

Other relevant WHO literature on health education

Principles and methods of health education. Report on a WHO Working Group, Dresden, 24-28 October, 1977. Copenhagen, WHO Regional Office for Europe, 1979 (EURO Reports and Studies, No. 11).

Webb JKG. *Health education for school-age children. The child-to-child programme.* Geneva, World Health Organization 1985.

Dowling MAC, Ritson R. *Learning materials for health workers.* WHO Chronicle, 1985, **39**(5):171–175.

New approaches to health education in primary health care. Report of a WHO Expert Committee. Geneva, World Health Organization, 1983 (WHO Technical Report Series, No. 690).

Research in health education. Report of a WHO Scientific Group. Geneva, World Health Organization, 1969 (WHO Technical Report Series, No. 432).

Teacher preparation for health education. Report of a Joint WHO/UNESCO Expert Committee. Geneva, World Health Organization, 1960 (WHO Technical Report Series, No. 193).

Bury JA et al. *Training and research in public health. Policy perspectives for a new public health.* Copenhagen, WHO Regional Office for Europe, 1994.

Comprehensive school health education: suggested guidelines for action. Geneva, World Health Organization, 1992.

Abbat FR. *Teaching for better learning. A guide for teachers of primary health care staff.* 2nd Edition. Geneva, World Health Organization, 1992.

Appendix 1

This annex is reproduced from *Foodborne disease: a focus for health education* (© World Health Organization, 1999). Applications and enquiries to reproduce or translate this annex should be addressed to the Office of Publications, Wold Health Organization, Geneva, Switzerland.

Causative agents of foodborne illness

The following tables provide concise information about the epidemiology of foodborne diseases and how they can be prevented. The tables give the name (and alternative names) of foodborne illnesses, together with the following information about each of them:

- the code by which the illness is classified in the International classification of diseases, 9th and 10th revisions (ICD-9 and ICD-10);
- the etiological agent that cause the illness;
- the main characteristics of the etiological agent;
- the incubation period of the illness;
- the symptoms;
- the sequelae that may result from the illness;
- the duration of the illness;
- the reservoir or source of the etiological agent;
- the mode of transmission of the agent, together with examples of foods that have been involved in outbreaks;
- measures that can be taken to control/prevent the spread of the etiological agent (by industry, by professional and domestic food handlers, and by consumers);
- the occurrence of the illness, as indicated by +(less 1 case per 100 000 population), ++ (1-100 cases per 100 000 population) and +++ (over 100 case per 100 000 population);
- the geographical occurrence of the illness;
- other details about the nature of the illness or about the agent that causes it.

The diseases are listed in alphabetical order by type of pathogen, with bacteria first, then viruses and then parasites (protozoa, nematodes, cestodes, and trematodes).

Appendix

The following bibliographical sources have been used in the preparation of this Appendix:

Benenson AS, ed. *Control of Communicable Diseases Manual: an official report of the American Public Health Association.* 16th ed. Washington DC, American Public Health Association, 1995.

Foodborne pathogens: risk and consequences. Task force report. Ames, USA Council of Agricultural Science and Technology, 1994.

Hobbs B, Roberts D. *Food Poisoning and Food Hygiene.* 6th ed. London, Edward Arnold, 1993.

Management of Outbreaks of Foodborne Illness. London, Department of Health, 1994.

Motarjemi Y, Käferstein, FK. Global Estimation of foodborne diseases. *World health statistics quarterly*, 1997 **50**(1/2): 5-11.

Quevedo F, Thakur AS. *Foodborne Parasitic Diseases.* Washington DC, Pan American Health Organization, 1990, (Series of scientific and technical monographs Number 12, Rev.1).

Type of illness	*Aeromonas* enteritis
Etiological agent	**Bacteria**: *Aeromonas hydrophila*.
Characteristics of the agent	Gram-negative, motile, non-spore-forming, facultatively anaerobic, straight or curved rods that will not grow in 4–5% salt or at pH < 6. Optimum growth temperature is 28 °C, but growth may occur at lower temperatures, down to 4 °C. Many strains have the ability to grow over a wide pH range (4–10) under otherwise optimal conditions.
Incubation period	24–48 hours.
Symptoms	Watery stools, stomach cramps, mild fever and vomiting.
Sequelae	Bronchopneumonia, cholecystitis.
Duration	Days–weeks.
Reservoir/source	A common organism found in aquatic environments that has been isolated from a wide range of foods.
Mode of transmission and example of foods involved in outbreaks	Seafood (fish, shrimp, oysters), snails, drinking water.
Specific control measures	*Industrial*: treatment and disinfection of water supplies, food irradiation. *Food service establishment/household*: thorough cooking of food, no long-term refrigeration of ready-to-eat foods.
Occurrence	Worldwide. Sporadic outbreaks have been reported from Africa, Australia, Europe, Japan and North America. Estimated rate of occurrence: unknown.
Other comments	Opportunistic pathogen.

Type of illness	***Bacillus cereus* gastroenteritis** a) Diarrhoeal syndrome b) Emetic syndrome
ICD code	ICD-9: 005.8 ICD-10: A05.4
Etiological agent	**Bacterial toxin:** a) *Bacillus cereus* diarrhoeal toxin causing toxic infection due to production of heat-labile toxins either in the gut or in food. b) *Bacillus cereus* emetic toxin causing intoxication due to heat-stable toxins produced in food.
Characteristics of the agent	Gram-positive, facultatively anaerobic, motile rods which produce heat-resistant spores; generally mesophilic, growing between 10 °C and 50 °C, with the optimum at 28–37 °C (there are, however, psychrotrophic strains which grow at 4 °C). They will grow in a pH range of 4.3–9.3 and water activity (a_w) above 0.92. Spores are moderately heat-resistant, and survive freezing and drying. Some strains require heat activation for spores to germinate and outgrow.
Incubation period	a) Diarrhoeal syndrome: 8–16 hours. b) Emetic syndrome: 1–5 hours.
Symptoms	a) Diarrhoeal syndrome: acute diarrhoea, nausea and abdominal pain. b) Emetic syndrome: acute nausea, vomiting and abdominal pain and sometimes diarrhoea.
Duration	a) Diarrhoeal syndrome: 24–36 hours. b) Emetic syndrome: 24–36 hours.
Reservoir/source	Widely distributed in nature (soil).
Mode of transmission and example of foods involved in outbreaks	Ingestion of food that has been stored at ambient temperatures after cooking, permitting the growth of bacterial spores and production of toxin. Many outbreaks (particularly those of emetic syndrome) are associated with cooked or fried rice that has been kept at ambient temperature. Examples of foods involved include starchy products, such as boiled or fried rice, spices, dried foods, milk and dairy products, vegetable dishes and sauces.
Specific control measures	*Food service establishment/household*: Effective temperature control to prevent spore germination and growth: food storage at >60 °C or properly refrigerated at <10 °C until use, unless other factors such as pH or a_w are such as to prevent growth; When refrigeration facilities are not available, cook only quantities required for immediate consumption. Toxins associated with emetic syndrome are heat-resistant and reheating, including stir frying, will not destroy them.
Occurrence	Worldwide. Estimated rate of occurrence: ++/+++.

Type of illness	**Botulism**
ICD code	ICD-9: 005.1 ICD-10: A05.1
Etiological agent	**Bacterial toxin**: toxins of *Clostridium botulinum*.
Characteristics of the agent	Gram-positive, spore-forming, obligately anaerobic, motile rods which produce seven potent neurotoxins A–G; only A, B, E, and, infrequently F have been associated with human disease (*Clostridium botulinum*). Group G is named *Clostridium argentinense*. The toxins are potentially lethal in very small doses. They act by binding at the neuromuscular junction, blocking nerve transmission and causing flaccid paralysis. Proteolytic strains of *C. botulinum* producing toxin types A, B and F are mesophilic, growing over the range 10–50 °C. Non-proteolytic strains producing toxin types B, E and F are psychrotrophic and can grow at temperatures as low as 3.3 °C. Minimum a_w for growth is 0.93–0.94 and minimum pH for growth is 4.6 (proteolytic strains) or 5.0 (non-proteolytic strains). The toxin is heat-labile and can be destroyed by adequate heat treatment (boiling for 15 minutes). Spores are resistant to normal cooking temperatures, and survive drying and freezing.
Incubation period	12–36 hours although may range from a few hours to 8 days.
Symptoms	Vomiting, abdominal pain, fatigue, muscle weakness, headache, dizziness, ocular disturbance (blurred or double vision, dilated pupils, unreactive to light), constipation, dry mouth and difficulty in swallowing and speaking, and ultimately paralysis and respiratory or heart failure.
Duration	From days up to 8 months; treatment is normally the rapid administration of antitoxin, alkaline stomach washing and mechanical respiratory support.
Reservoir/source	Soil, marine and freshwater sediments and the intestinal tracts of fish, animals, birds and insects.
Mode of transmission and example of foods involved in outbreaks	Ingestion of toxin pre-formed in the food. This may occur when raw or under-processed foods are stored in conditions (temperature, a_w, pH and atmosphere) allowing growth of the organism. Most outbreaks are due to faulty preservation of food (particularly in homes or cottage industries), e.g. canning, fermentation, curing, or smoking, acid or oil preservation. Examples of foods involved include vegetables, condiments (e.g. pepper), fish and fish products (type E), meat and meat products. Several outbreaks have occurred as a result of consumption of uneviscerated fish, garlic in oil and baked potatoes. Honey is suspected as a mode of transmission of infant botulism.
Specific control mesures	The toxin is destroyed by boiling, however spores require a much higher temperature. *Industrial*: heat sterilization; use of nitrites in pasteurized meat. *Food service establishment/household*: acid-preservation of food at a low pH (<4.6); thorough cooking of home-canned food (boil and stir for 15 minutes); refrigerated storage of food, particularly vacuum-packed, fresh or lightly cured/smoked food. *Consumers* should: avoid giving honey or foods containing honey to infants; discard swollen cans.
Occurrence	Worldwide; particularly frequent among Alaskan populations due to faulty fermentation. Estimated rate of occurrence: +.
Other comments	Case–fatality rate in industrialized countries is in the range 5–10%.

Type of illness	**Brucellosis (undulant fever)**
ICD code	ICD-9: 023 ICD-10: A23
Etiological agent	**Bacteria:** a) *Brucella abortus* b) *Brucella melitensis* c) *Brucella suis*
Characteristics of the agent	Gram-negative, aerobic, non-spore-forming, short, oval non-motile rods which grow optimally at 37 °C; heat-labile. Optimum pH for growth: 6.6–7.4.
Incubation period	Variable, from a few days to several weeks or months.
Symptoms	Continuous, intermittent or irregular fever, lassitude, sweat, headache, chills, constipation, body pain, weight loss and anorexia.
Sequelae	Bouts of fever, osteoarticular complications in 20–60% of cases, sacroiliitis, genitourinary complications (including orchitis, epididymitis, sexual impotence), cardiovascular and neurological conditions, insomnia, depression.
Duration	Weeks.
Reservoir/source	Cows, goats, pigs, sheep. a) *Brucella abortus*: cows. b) *Brucella melitensis*: sheep and goats. c) *Brucella suis*: pigs.
Mode of transmission and example of foods involved in outbreaks	Contracted principally from close association with infected animals and therefore an occupational disease of farmers, herdsmen, veterinarians and slaughterhouse workers. It can also be contracted by consumption of milk usually goat's or sheep's milk), and products made from unpasteurized milk, e.g. fresh goat cheese.
Specific control measures	*Industrial*: heat treatment of milk (pasteurization or sterilization), use of pasteurized milk for cheese production, ageing cheese for at least 90 days. *Food service establishment/household*: heat treatment of milk (boiling). *Other*: vaccination of animals; eradication of diseased animals (testing and slaughtering). *Consumers* should avoid eating/drinking raw milk and eating cheese made with raw milk.
Occurrence	Worldwide, with the exception of parts of northern Europe where it occurs rarely. Incidence in North America is decreasing. Currently reported incidence in the USA is below 120 cases per year. Prevalent in eastern Mediterranean areas, southern Europe, North and East Africa, Central and Southern Asia (India), Central and South America (e.g. Mexico). Estimated rate of occurrence depending on the region: + or ++.
Other comments	The disease is often unrecognized and unreported. Susceptible to antibiotic treatment. Case–fatality rate may be up to 2% if the disease is untreated.

Type of illness	**Campylobacteriosis**
ICD code	ICD-9: 008.4 ICD-0: A04.5
Etiological agent	**Bacteria:** *Campylobacter jejuni* and *Campylobacter coli*.
Characteristics of the agent	Gram-negative, non-spore-forming, curved or spiral, motile rods which are sensitive to oxygen and grow best at low oxygen levels in the presence of carbon dioxide. Optimum pH 6.5–7.5. They will not grow below 28–30 °C, grow optimally at 42–45 °C and are very sensitive to heat, salt, reduced pH levels (<6.5) and dry conditions. The organism survives better in cold conditions than ambient temperature.
Incubation period	1–11 days, most commonly 2–5 days.
Symptoms	Fever, severe abdominal pain, nausea, and diarrhoea which can vary from slight to profuse watery diarrhoea sometimes containing blood or mucus.
Sequelae	Sequelae may occur in 2–10% of cases. These include reactive arthritis, Guillain–Barré syndrome, haemolytic uraemic syndrome, meningitis, pancreatitis, cholecystitis, colitis, endocarditis, erythema nodosum.
Duration	Up to 10 days; excretion of the organism can continue for 2–3 weeks.
Reservoir/source	Domestic animals (cats, dogs), livestock (pigs, cattle, sheep), birds (poultry), polluted water.
Mode of transmission and example of foods involved in outbreaks	Main food sources are raw milk and raw or undercooked poultry. The bacteria can be spread to other foods by cross-contamination, or contamination with untreated water, contact with animals and birds. Other sources of transmission are contact with live can also occur during the infectious period which ranges from several days to several weeks. Examples of foods involved include raw milk, poultry, beef, pork and drinking-water.
Specific control measures	*Industrial:* heat treatment (pasteurization/sterilization of milk); hygienic slaughter and processing procedures, irradiation of meat and poultry; treatment of water. *Food service establishment/household:* heat treatment of milk (boiling); thorough cooking of all meat; washing of salads; prevention of cross-contamination of contact surfaces; personal hygiene in food preparation (hand-washing after contact with animals); keeping pets away from food-handling areas. *Consumers* should avoid eating raw or partially-cooked poultry and drinking raw milk.
Occurrence	Worldwide. This is one of the most frequently reported foodborne diseases in industrialized countries. In developing countries it is a major cause of infant and traveller's diarrhoea. Some 10–15% of cases of diarrhoeal disease in children seen at treatment centres are caused by *Campylobacter spp*. Estimated rate of occurrence: ++/+++ in industrialized and developing countries respectively.
Other comments	Many infections are asymptomatic. Infected individuals not treated with antibiotics may excrete the organisms for as long as 2–7 weeks. Infection is sometimes misdiagnosed as appendicitis. More sporadic cases occur in the warmer months. The case–fatality rate in industrialized countries is about 0.05%. Infants and young children are the most susceptible.

Appendix

Type of illness	**Cholera**
ICD code	ICD-9: 001 ICD-10: A00
Etiological agent	**Bacteria**: *Vibrio cholerae* O1 (enterotoxin in the gut). Two biotypes are distinguished: classical and eltor. These are further divided in Ogawa and Inaba serotypes. Also, *Vibrio cholerae* O139.
Characteristics of the agent	Gram-negative, facultatively anaerobic, motile, non-spore-forming rods which grow at 18–42 °C and optimally at 37 °C. Will grow down to a_w 0.97 and over a pH range of 6–11; optimum pH is 7.6. Growth is stimulated by salinity levels of around 3% but is prevented at 6%. They are resistant to freezing but sensitive to heat and acid and may survive for some days on fruit and vegetables. *V. cholerae* is non-invasive and diarrhoea is mediated by cholera-toxin formed in the gut.
Incubation period	1–3 days.
Symptoms	Profuse watery diarrhoea, which can lead to severe dehydration, collapse and death within a few hours unless lost fluid and salt are replaced; abdominal pain and vomiting.
Duration	Up to 7 days.
Reservoir/source	Humans. *V. cholerae* is often found in aquatic environments and is part of the normal flora in brackish water and estuaries.
Mode of transmission and example of foods involved in outbreaks	Food and water contaminated through contact with faecal matter or infected food handlers. Contamination of vegetables may occur through sewage or wastewater used for irrigation. Person-to-person transmission through the faecal–oral route is also an important mode of transmission. Examples of foods involved include seafood, vegetables, cooked rice, and ice.
Specific control measures	*Industrial*: control measures include safe disposal of excreta and sewage/wastewater; treatment of drinking-water, e.g. chlorination; irradiation, heat treatment of foods, e.g. canning. *Food service establishment/household*: personal hygiene (washing hands with soap and water); thorough cooking of food and careful washing of fruit and vegetables; boiling drinking-water when safe water is not available. *Consumers* should avoid eating raw seafood. In some countries, travellers may need to be vaccinated.
Occurrence	Africa, Asia, parts of Europe and Latin America. In most industrialized countries, reported cholera cases are imported by travellers, or occur as a result of import of food by travellers. Estimated rate of occurrence: in industrialized countries it occurs rarely and is mainly imported. In Africa and Central and South America, +/++, and in other parts of the world +.
Other comments	In endemic areas, cholera occurs mainly in children because of lack of prior immunity; in epidemics children and adults are equally susceptible. Case–fatality rate can be less than 1% with adequate treatment; in untreated cases, the case–fatality rate may exceed 50%.

Type of illness	*Clostridium perfringens* enteritis
ICD code	ICD-9: 005.2 ICD-10: A05.2
Etiological agent	**Bacteria** *Clostridium perfringens* (produces enterotoxin in the gut) also known as *Clostridium welchii*.
Characteristics of the agent	Gram-positive, non-motile, anaerobic, spore-forming rods that will grow in the temperature range 12–50 °C, although very slowly below 20 °C. They grow extremely quickly at optimum temperature 43–47 °C. Optimum pH is between 6 and 7, but growth will occur as low as pH 5. Lowest a_w supporting growth is 0.95.
Incubation period	8–24 hours.
Symptoms	Abdominal pain and diarrhoea. Vomiting and fever are rare.
Duration	1–2 days
Reservoir/source	Soil, sewage, dust, faeces of animals and humans, animal-origin feedstuffs.
Mode of transmission and example of foods involved in outbreaks	Illness is usually caused by cooked meat and poultry dishes subject to time–temperature abuse. The dish has usually been left too long at ambient temperature for cooling before storage, or cooled inadequately. This allows spores surviving the cooking process to germinate and grow, producing large numbers of vegetative cells. If the dish is not reheated sufficiently before consumption to kill the vegetative cells then illness can result. Examples of foods involved include meat and poultry (boiled, stewed or casseroled).
Specific control measures	*Food service establishment/household:* adequate cooling and cool storage of cooked products: meat based sauces and large pieces of meat should be cooled to <10°C within 2–3 hours; thorough reheating of stored food before consumption; preparation of quantities as required when there is no available refrigeration.
Occurrence	Worldwide. Estimated rate of occurrence: ++/+++.
Other comments	Case–fatality rate in industrialized countries is very low at <0.1%.

Type of illness	*Escherichia coli* infections
ICD code	ICD-9: 008.0 ICD-10: A04.0–A04.3 (EPEC: A04.0; ETEC: A04.1, EIEC: A04.2; EHEC: A04.3)
Etiological agent	**Bacteria**: a) *E. coli* enteropathogenic (EPEC). b) *E. coli* enterotoxigenic (ETEC) produces two types of enterotoxins: a heat-labile toxin (LT) and a heat-stable toxin (ST). c) *E. coli* enteroinvasive (EIEC). d) *E. coli* enterohaemorrhagic (EHEC) or verocytotoxin-producing *E. coli* (VTEC).
Characteristics of the agent	Gram-negative, non-spore-forming, facultatively anaerobic rods, which belong to the family Enterobacteriaceae. Typically mesophile, the bacteria will grow from about 7–10 °C up to 50 °C, with the optimum at 37 °C; in a pH range of 4.4–8.5. Minimum a_w for growth is 0.95. Most *E. coli* are harmless inhabitants of the gut of humans and other warm-blooded animals, however the strains mentioned above may cause diseases. EHEC is more acid-resistant than other *E. coli*.
Incubation period	a) EPEC: 1–6 days; as short as 12–36 hours. b) ETEC: 1–3 days; as short as 10–12 hours. c) EIEC: 1–3 days; as short as 10–18 hours. d) EHEC: 3–8 days, with a median of 4 days.
Symptoms	a) EPEC infection: enteropathogenic *E. coli* adhere to the mucosa and change its absorption capacity causing vomiting, diarrhoea, abdominal pain, and fever. b) ETEC infection: health effects are mediated by enterotoxins. Symptoms include diarrhoea (ranging from mild afebrile diarrhoea to a severe, cholera-like syndrome of profuse diarrhoea without blood or mucus), abdominal cramps and vomiting, sometimes leading to dehydration and shock. c) EIEC infection: inflammatory disease of the gut mucosa and submucosa caused by the invasion and multiplication of EIEC in the epithelial cells of the colon. Symptoms include fever, severe abdominal pain, vomiting and watery diarrhoea (in <10% of cases stools may become bloody and may contain mucous). d) EHEC infection: abdominal cramps, watery diarrhoea that may develop into bloody diarrhoea (haemorrhagic colitis). Fever and vomiting may also occur.
Sequelae	EPEC, ETEC, EIEC infections are an underlying factor of malnutrition in infants and children in developing countries. EHEC infections may result in life-threatening complications, such as haemolytic uraemic syndrome (HUS): in up to 10% of patients, particularly, young children and the elderly. HUS is characterized by acute renal failure, haemolytic anaemia and thrombocytopenia. Other sequelae include erythema nodosum and thrombotic thrombocytopenic purpura.
Duration	a) EPEC: days–weeks. b) ETEC: up to 5 days. c) EIEC: days–weeks. d) EHEC: days–weeks.
Reservoir/source	Humans are the main reservoir for EPEC, ETEC, EIEC. The reservoir for EHEC is mainly cattle.

Mode of transmission and example of foods involved in outbreaks	EPEC, ETEC, EIEC infections: consumption of food and water contaminated with faecal matter. Time–temperature abuse of such food increases the risk of illness. Up to 25% of infections in infants and young children in developing countries are due to *E. coli*, in particular ETEC and EPEC, which are observed in 10–20 % and 1–5 % of cases at treatment centres respectively. ETEC is also a major cause of traveller's diarrhoea in developing countries. EHEC infection is transmitted mainly through consumption of foods such as raw or undercooked ground-meat products, and raw milk, from infected animals. Faecal contamination of water and other foods, as well as cross-contamination during food preparation, will also lead to infection. Examples of foods involved include ground (minced) meat, raw milk, and vegetables. Secondary transmission (person-to-person) may also occur during the period of excretion of the pathogen which is less than a week for adults but up to 3 weeks in one-third of children affected.
Specific control measures	*Industrial*: treatment of drinking water, and an effective sewage disposal system. *Food service establishment/household*: specific control measures based on prevention of direct and indirect contamination of food and water with faecal matter; thorough cooking and reheating of food; and good personal hygiene. For EHEC infection, control measures include: *Industrial*: irradiation of meat, or thorough heat processing of meat; pasteurization/sterilization of milk; treatment of wastewater used for irrigation. *Food service establishment/household*: thorough cooking of meat, boiling of milk or use of pasteurized milk; separation of raw and cooked foods, hand-washing before preparation of food. *Consumers* should avoid eating raw or partially cooked meat and poultry and drinking raw milk.
Occurrence	Worldwide. *E. coli* infections are highly prevalent in developing countries where the estimated rate of occurrence is +++. EHEC infections are mainly reported in Argentina, Chile, Europe (France, Germany, Italy, Sweden, UK), Japan and North America.
Other comments	The case–fatality rate of EPEC, ETEC, EIEC infections in industrialized countries is estimated to be less than 0.1%. The case–fatality rate of EHEC infection is about 2%. The fatality rate of *E. coli* infections in infants and children is much higher in developing countries. Children and the elderly are particularly vulnerable to this infection and may suffer more severely. The majority of cases of EHEC infections are reported in summer.

Type of illness	Listeriosis
ICD code	ICD-9: 027 ICD-10: A32
Etiological agent	**Bacteria**: *Listeria monocytogenes*.
Characteristics of the agent	Gram-positive, non-spore-forming, facultatively anaerobic, rods. Psychrotrophic, capable of growing in a temperature range of 3–42 °C., but optimally at about 30-35 °C. The pH range for growth is 5.0–9. Minimum pH and a_w for growth are 4.4 and 0.92 respectively. The bacteria are able to grow in the presence of 10% salt.
Incubation period	A few days to several weeks.
Symptoms	Influenza-like symptoms such as fever, headache and occasionally gastrointestinal symptoms.
Sequelae	Meningoencephalitis and/or septicaemia in newborns and adults and abortion in pregnant women. The onset of meningoencephalitis (rare in pregnant women) may be sudden with fever, intense headaches, nausea, vomiting and signs of meningeal irritation. Delirium and coma may appear early; occasionally there is collapse and shock.
Duration	Days–weeks.
Reservoir/source	Water, soil, sewage, sludge, decaying vegetables, silage and faeces of numerous wild and domestic animals. Other sources may be infected animals and people.
Mode of transmission and example of foods involved in outbreaks	A substantial proportion of cases of listeriosis are foodborne. Examples of foods involved include raw milk, soft cheese, meat-based paste, jellied pork tongue, raw vegetables and coleslaw.
Specific control measures	*Industrial:* heat treatment of milk (pasteurization, sterilization) with measures to ensure reduction of processing contamination risks. For ready-to-eat high-risk processed foods, reduction of all cross-contamination risks after processing. *Food service establishment/household:* use of pasteurized or heat-treated (boiling) milk and products made from pasteurized or heat-treated milk; refrigeration of perishable foods and consumption within a short space of time. Pre-cooked refrigerated foods should be thoroughly reheated before consumption. Avoidance of certain high risk foods e.g. soft cheese, ready-to-eat meat such as paté, and raw milk and raw milk products during pregnancy. *Consumers*, particularly pregnant women and other vulnerable individuals should avoid eating raw foods of animal origin, e.g. raw meat, raw milk. Pregnant women should also avoid foods which support growth of *Listeria*, e.g. soft cheese, pre-prepared salad, cold, smoked or raw seafood, paté.
Ocurrence	Estimated rate of occurrence: +. The majority of cases reported have been from Europe, North America and the islands of the Pacific.
Other comments	The most severe form of illness occurs in fetuses and neonates, the elderly and those who are immunocompromised. About one-third of clinical cases occur in the newborn. In adults infection occurs mainly in those aged 40 or over. Transplacental fetal infection may lead to abortion or stillbirth. Asymptomatic infection may occur at all ages. Infected individuals may shed the organisms in their stools for several months. Case–fatality rate is up to 30%; in patients who have not received adequate treatment the case–fatality rate may be as high as 70%. Pregnant women and fetuses, the elderly, and immunocompromised individuals, including those receiving treatments for cancer, are the most susceptible.

Type of illness	**Salmonellosis**
ICD code	ICD-9: 003 ICD-10: A02.0
Etiological agent	**Bacteria**: non-typhoid *Salmonella* serotypes.
Characteristics of the agent	Gram-negative, mesophilic, facultatively anaerobic, motile, non-spore-forming rods. Growth can occur between 5 °C and 47 °C. Optimum growth occurs at 37 °C. Minimum pH and a_w for growth are 4 and 0.95 respectively.
Incubation period	6–48 hours, occasionally up to 4 days.
Symptoms	The principal symptoms are fever, headache, nausea, vomiting, abdominal pain and diarrhoea.
Sequelae	Reactive arthritis, septicaemia, aortitis, cholecystitis, colitis, meningitis, myocarditis, osteomyelitis, pancreatitis, Reiter disease, rheumatoid syndromes.
Duration	Usually a few days to 1 week, but sometimes infection may last up to 3 weeks.
Reservoir/source	A wide range of domestic and wild animals, including poultry, pigs, cattle, rodents, iguanas, pets such as tortoises, turtles, chicks, dogs and cats. Also humans, i.e. patients and convalescent carriers.
Mode of transmission and example of foods involved in outbreaks	The main route of transmission is by ingestion of the organisms in food (milk, meat, poultry, eggs) derived from infected food animals. Food can also be contaminated by infected food handlers, pets and pests, or by cross-contamination owing to poor hygiene. Contamination of food and water may also occur from the faeces of an infected animal or person. Problems caused by initial contamination may be exacerbated by prolonged storage at temperatures at which the organism may grow. Direct person-to-person transmission may also occur during the course of the infection. Examples of foods involved include unpasteurized milk, raw eggs, poultry, meat, spices, salads, chocolate.
Specific control measures	*Industrial:* effective heat-processing of foods of animal origin including pasteurization of milk and eggs; irradiation of meat and poultry. *Food service establishment/household:* safe food preparation practices, including thorough cooking and reheating of food and boiling of milk; adequate refrigeration; prevention of cross-contamination, cleaning and disinfection of food preparation surfaces; exclusion of pets and other animals from food-handling areas. *Consumers*, particularly vulnerable groups, should avoid raw and undercooked meat and poultry, as well as raw milk and raw eggs and foods containing raw eggs.
Occurrence	Worldwide. Estimated rate of occurrence: ++ /+++. A drastic increase in incidence of salmonellosis, due particularly to S. Enteritidis, has occurred during the past two decades in Europe, North America, and some other countries. In Europe and North America, contaminated eggs and poultry have been the major source of infection.
Other comments	General susceptibility is increased by achlorhydria, antacid therapy, immunosuppressive therapy and other debilitating conditions, including malnutrition. The severity of the illness is related to serotype, the number of organisms ingested and host factors. Case–fatality rate is less than 1% in industrialized countries. Symptomless excretion of the organism can continue for several weeks or, in some cases, months.

Type of illness	**Shigellosis (or bacillary dysentery)**
ICD code	ICD-9: 004 ICD-10: A03
Etiological agent	**Bacteria:** *Shigella dysenteriae, S. flexneri, S. boydii, S. sonnei.*
Characteristics of the agent	Gram-negative, non-motile, non-spore-forming, facultatively anaerobic rods. Typically mesophilic: growing between 10 °C and 45 °C and optimally at 37 °C. The bacteria grow best in the pH range 6–8 and do not survive below pH 4.5. The minimum a_w for growth is 0.97.
Incubation period	1–3 days, up to 1 week for *S. dysenteriae*.
Symptoms	Abdominal pain, vomiting, fever accompanied by diarrhoea that can range from watery (*S. sonnei*) to a dysenteric syndrome of bloody stools containing mucus and pus (*Sh. dysenteriae* and, to a lesser extent, *S. flexneri* and *S. boydii*).
Sequelae	In 2–3% of cases these may be: haemolytic uraemic syndrome, erythema nodosum, Reiter disease, splenic abscesses, synovitis.
Duration	A few days to a few weeks.
Reservoir/source	Humans.
Mode of transmission and example of foods involved in outbreaks	Food and water contaminated with faecal matter. Person-to-person transmission through the faecal–oral route is an important mode of transmission. Food can be contaminated by food handlers with poor personal hygiene or by use of sewage/wastewater for fertilization. Examples of foods involved include uncooked foods that have received extensive handling such as mixed salads and vegetables; water and raw milk.
Specific control measures	*Industrial:* treatment of drinking water and an effective sewage disposal system. *Food service establishment/household:* safe food preparation practices including careful hand-washing with soap and water, thorough cooking and reheating of food prior to consumption, disinfection of food preparation surfaces and thorough washing of all fruit and vegetables.
Occurrence	Worldwide, with a higher prevalence in developing countries. Shigellosis is a major cause of diarrhoea in infants and children under the age of 5 years, and constitutes 5–15% of diarrhoeal disease cases seen at treatment centres. *S. dysenteriae* type 1 has been responsible for large epidemics of severe dysentery in Central America and recently Central Africa and southern Asia. Depending on the degree of development the estimated rate of occurrence may vary between + and +++.
Other comments	In developing countries, *S. flexneri* is the most common cause of infection. However, *S. dysenteriae* type 1, occurring in epidemic regions, causes the most severe disease. In industrialized countries, *S. sonnei* is the most common species isolated, and milder illness is the norm. The disease is more severe in young children than in adults among whom many infections may be asymptomatic. The elderly and those suffering from malnutrition are particularly susceptible and may develop severe symptoms or even die. Travellers are particularly at risk. Case–fatality rate in industrialized countries is low and estimated at 0.1%.

Type of illness	***Staphylococcus aureus* intoxication**
ICD code	ICD-9: 005.0 ICD-10: A05.0
Etiological agent	**Bacterial toxin:** *Staphylococcus aureus* enterotoxin.
Characteristics of the agent	Gram-positive, non-motile, non-spore-forming facultatively anaerobic cocci. Growth temperature is between 7 °C and 48 °C, with an optimum of about 37°C. They grow in a pH range of 4–9.3. Optimum pH is 7.0–7.5. The range over which enterotoxin is produced is narrower, with little toxin production below pH 6.0. Growth will occur down to an a_w of 0.83, but toxin production does not occur below 0.86. This is the most resistant bacterial pathogen with regard to decreased water activity. Intoxication is caused by a toxin which is formed in the food. The toxin is relatively heat-stable and can survive boiling for more than an hour. It is therefore possible for well-cooked food to cause illness but not contain any viable *S. aureus* cells.
Incubation period	2–6 hours
Symptoms	An intoxication, sometimes of abrupt and violent onset. Severe nausea, cramps, vomiting and prostration, sometimes accompanied by diarrhoea.
Duration	About 2 days.
Reservoir/source	Humans (skin, nose, throat). *S. aureus* is carried by about 25–40 % of the healthy population.
Mode of transmission and example of foods involved in outbreaks	Consumption of foods containing the toxin. Foods are contaminated by food handlers. If storage conditions are inadequate, the bacteria may multiply to produce toxin. Intoxication is often associated with cooked food, e.g. meat, where competitive bacteria have been destroyed. Examples of foods involved include prepared foods subject to handling in their preparation (ham, chicken and egg salads, cream-filled products, ice-cream, cheese).
Specific control measures	*Food service establishment/household*: Exclusion of food handlers with visibly infected skin lesions (boils, cuts etc) from work; thorough personal hygiene of workers; prevention of time–temperature abuse in handling cooked/ready-to-eat foods.
Occurrence	Worldwide. The estimated rate of occurrence varies between ++ and +++ depending on conditions of food hygiene.
Other comments	Case–fatality rate is estimated at less than 0.02%.

Type of illness	**Typhoid and paratyphoid fevers**
ICD code	ICD-9: 002.0 and 002.1–002.9 ICD-10: A01.0 and A01.1–A01.4
Etiological agent	**Bacteria:** *Salmonella* Typhi and *Salmonella* Paratyphi types A–C.
Characteristics of the agent	As for non-typhoid salmonellae, except minimum growth pH is higher (4.9).
Incubation period	10–20 days with a range of 3 days to 8 weeks.
Symptoms	Systemic infections characterized by high fever, abdominal pains, headache, vomiting, diarrhoea followed by constipation, rashes and other symptoms of generalized infection.
Sequelae	Haemolytic anaemia.
Duration	Several weeks to months.
Reservoir/source	Humans.
Mode of transmission and example of foods involved in outbreaks	Ingestion of food and water contaminated with faecal matter. Food handlers carrying the pathogen may be an important source of food contamination. Secondary transmission may also occur. Examples of foods involved include prepared foods, dairy products (e.g. raw milk), meat products, shellfish, vegetables, salads.
Specific control measures	*Industrial:* treatment of drinking water, and an effective sewage disposal system. *Food service establishment/household:* safe food preparation practices including careful hand-washing with soap and water, thorough cooking and reheating of food prior to consumption, disinfection of food preparation surfaces and thorough washing of all fruit and vegetables.
Occurrence	Predominantly in developing countries where the estimated rate of occurrence is ++. In industrialized countries the estimated rate of occurrence is +.
Other comments	Excretion of the organism may occur after recovery or by asymptomatic carriers, and this may be lifelong unless treated. Case–fatality rate is estimated at about 6% in industrialized countries.

Type of illness	*Vibrio parahaemolyticus* gastroenteritis
ICD code	ICD-9: 005.4 ICD-10: A.05.3
Etiological agent	**Bacteria**: *Vibrio parahaemolyticus*
Characteristics of the agent	Basic characteristics are the same as for *V. cholerae*. *V. parahaemolyticus* differs in that it is halophilic and will grow at salt levels up to 8% and with a minimum a_w of 0.94. Growth is optimal and very fast at 37 °C (doubling time about 10 minutes) and will occur down to around 10 °C. *V. parahaemolyticus* is more sensitive to extremes of temperature than *V. cholerae* and will die at chill temperatures.
Incubation period	Often 9–25 hours, up to 3 days
Symptoms	Profuse watery diarrhoea free from blood or mucus, abdominal pain, vomiting, and fever. A dysenteric syndrome has been reported from some countries, particularly Japan.
Sequelae	Septicaemia.
Duration	Up to 8 days.
Reservoir/source	Natural habitat is coastal seawater and estuarine brackish waters above 15 °C and marine fish and shellfish.
Mode of transmission and example of foods involved in outbreaks	Mainly consumption of raw or undercooked fish and fishery products, or cooked foods subject to cross-contamination from raw fish.
Specific control measures	*Food service establishment/household*: thorough heat treatment of seafood; rapid chilling; prevention of cross-contamination from raw seafood products to other foods or preparation surfaces.
Occurrence	The illness has been reported primarily in countries in the western Pacific region and in particular Japan as well as south-east Asia and the USA. Estimated rate of occurrence: +/++.
Other comments	Case–fatality rate in industrialized countries is less than 1%.

Type of illness	*Vibrio vulnificus* infection
ICD code	ICD-9: 005.8 ICD-10: A05.8
Etiological agent	**Bacteria**: *Vibrio vulnificus*.
Characteristics of the agent	Gram-negative, non-spore-forming rods. Optimal temperature for growth is 37 °C.
Incubation period	12 hours–3 days.
Symptoms	Profuse diarrhoea with blood in stools; the organism is associated with wound infections and septicaemia which may originate from the gastrointestinal tract, or traumatized epithelial surfaces.
Sequelae	Produces septicaemia in persons with chronic liver diseases, chronic alcoholism, haemochromatosis, or those who are immunodepressed. Over 50% of patients with primary septicaemia may die; the fatality rate increases to 90% in hypotensive individuals.
Duration	Days–weeks.
Reservoir/source	Natural habitat is coastal or estuarine waters.
Mode of transmission and example of foods involved in outbreaks	All known cases are associated with seafood, particularly raw oysters.
Specific control measures	*Consumers*, particularly vulnerable groups including the elderly, those with underlying liver disease or immunodepressed through treatment or disease, and alcoholics, should not eat raw seafood.
Occurrence	Frequently in Europe, USA and the Western Pacific Region. Estimated rate of occurrence: +/++.
Other comments	Case–fatality rate can be as high as 40–60%.

Type of illness	**Yersiniosis**
ICD code	ICD-9: 027.8 ICD-10: A04.6
Etiological agent	**Bacteria**: *Yersinia enterocolitica*
Characteristics of the agent	Gram-negative, facultatively anaerobic, motile, non-spore-forming rods of the family Enterobacteriaceae. *Y. enterocolitica* is a psychrotroph capable of growing at temperatures between 0 °C and 44 °C, but optimally at 29 °C. Growth will occur in a pH range of 4.6–9.0, but optimally at pH 7–8. It will grow in media containing 5% salt but not 7% salt.
Incubation period	1–11 days (but usually 24–36 hours).
Symptoms	Abdominal pain, diarrhoea accompanied by a mild fever, and sometimes vomiting.
Sequelae	Sequelae are observed in 2–3% of cases: reactive arthritis, Reiter disease, eye complaints, cholangitis, erythema nodosum, septicaemia, hepatic and splenic abscesses, lymphadenitis, pneumonia, spondylitis.
Duration	Symptoms usually abate after 2–3 days; although they may continue in a milder form for 1–3 weeks.
Reservoir/source	A variety of animals, but pathogenic strains are most frequently isolated from pigs.
Mode of transmission and example of foods involved in outbreaks	Illness is transmitted through consumption of pork products (tongue, tonsils, gut), cured or uncured, as well as milk and milk products.
Specific control measures	*Food service establishment/household:* thorough cooking of pork products, and prevention of cross-contamination.
Occurrence	Northern Europe and Australia: estimated rate of occurrence: +/++; USA: estimated rate of occurrence: +.
Other comments	Untreated cases continue to excrete the organism for 2–3 months. The disease is often misdiagnosed as appendicitis. Case–fatality rate is 0.03%.

Type of illness	Poliomyelitis
ICD code	ICD-9: 045 ICD-10: A80
Etiological agent	**Virus**: Poliovirus; member of *Picornaviridae*.
Characteristics of the agent	Small round virus, which contains single-stranded RNA and can withstand acidity in the range of pH 3–5. The poliovirus infects the gastrointestinal tract and spreads to the regional nodes, and, in a minority of cases, to the nervous system.
Incubation period	3–14 days.
Symptoms	Poliomyelitis may be a transient viraemia characterized by fever and malaise. In a minority of cases, it may progress to a second stage of persistent viraemia where the virus invades the central nervous system causing varying degrees of paralysis and in some cases even death. Severe muscle pain and stiffness of the neck and back with or without flaccid paralysis are symptoms of the more severe illness. Flaccid paralysis occurs in less than 1% of poliovirus infections. Most often paralysis is in the legs, sometimes in the arms. Paralysis of the muscles used in respiration and/or swallowing is life threatening. The infection in young children is usually asymptomatic and confers immunity, but is more severe in older children and young adults.
Sequelae	Permanent paralysis.
Reservoir/source	Humans; most frequently people with no apparent symptoms of infection.
Mode of transmission and example of foods involved in outbreaks	Principally person-to-person, through the faecal–oral route. Food and drinking-water are potential modes of transmission where hygiene standards are low. In some instances, milk and other foodstuffs contaminated with faeces have been a vehicle for transmission.
Specific control measures	Vaccination. Specific control measures with regard to food include: *Industrial:* treatment of drinking-water, and an effective sewage disposal system. *Food service establishment/household:* safe food preparation practices including careful hand-washing with soap and water, thorough cooking and reheating of food prior to consumption and thorough washing of all fruit and vegetables.
Occurrence	Poliomyelitis has been almost entirely eradicated in industrialized countries and the Americas owing to effective immunization. It occurs in developing countries with an estimated rate of occurrence varying from + to ++, depending on immunization programmes.
Other comments	During the few days prior to, and following the onset of symptoms, the risk of transmission is greatest. Infants and children under 5 years of age are the most frequently affected. Immunization of the elderly is recommended, particularly when travelling abroad.

Type of illness	**Viral gastroenteritis**
ICD code	ICD-9: 008.8 ICD-10: A08
Etiological agent	**Virus**: a number of different viruses have been established as causes of gastroenteritis. These include adenoviruses, coronaviruses, rotaviruses, parvoviruses, caliciviruses and astroviruses. Those most commonly associated with foodborne outbreaks are described as small, round-structured viruses (SRSVs), which include Norwalk agent.
Characteristics of the agent	These viruses exhibit a range of biochemical and physical characteristics.
Incubation period	15–50 hours.
Symptoms	Diarrhoea and vomiting which is often severe and projectile with sudden onset.
Duration	2 days.
Reservoir/source	Humans.
Mode of transmission and example of foods involved in outbreaks	Gastroenteritis viruses are usually spread by the faecal–oral route. Food and drinking-water may be contaminated either at source when exposed to sewage/wastewater in the environment or used for irrigation, or by an infected food handler. Filter-feeding shellfish are the most common food contaminated at source, but a far wider range of different cooked and uncooked foods have been implicated in secondary contamination by food handlers.
Specific control measures	Hygienic sewage disposal, treatment of drinking-water, treatment of wastewater used for irrigation. Good personal hygiene (i.e. hand hygiene); abstinence from handling food when ill, especially when diarrhoea is present.
Occurrence	Worldwide. Estimated rate of occurrence for Rotavirus: ++/+++; and for other viral infections: +. Rotavirus infections constitute 15–25% of diarrhoeal disease cases identified in children seen at treatment centres in the developing countries.

Type of illness	**Viral hepatitis A**
ICD code	ICD-9: 070.1 ICD-10: B15
Etiological agent	**Virus**: Hepatitis A virus; member of *Picornaviridae*.
Characteristics of the agent	Small round virus, around 28 nm in diameter, containing single-stranded RNA. The virus multiplies in the gut epithelium before being carried by the blood to the liver. In the later part of incubation, the virus is shed in the faeces. Relatively acid-resistant.
Incubation period	2–6 weeks; usually about 25 days.
Symptoms	Early symptoms are loss of appetite, fever, malaise, abdominal discomfort, nausea and vomiting. These are followed by symptoms of liver damage such as passage of dark urine, pale stools and jaundice.
Sequelae	Liver disorders, particularly in older persons.
Duration	Varies in clinical severity: mild, with recovery within few weeks, to severe, lasting several months.
Reservoir/source	Humans: sewage and contaminated water.
Mode of transmission and example of foods involved in outbreaks	Spread through the faecal–oral route, primarily person-to-person. It can also be transmitted through food and water as a result of sewage contamination or infected food handlers. Risk of transmission is greatest during the second half of the incubation period until a few days after the appearance of jaundice. Examples of foods involved include: Shellfish, raw fruit and vegetables, bakery products.
Specific control measures	*Industrial*: treatment of water supply, safe sewage disposal. *Food service establishment/household*: good personal hygiene, in particular, thorough hand-washing with soap and water before handling foods and abstinence from handling food when infected; thorough cooking of shellfish. An effective vaccine is available, and vaccination of professional food handlers and travellers should be considered.
Occurrence	Worldwide. Estimated rate of occurrence: ++.
Other comments	There may be asymptomatic carriers. Infection in adults is most severe. In children it is often asymptomatic and confers immunity. Case–fatality rate is low, about 0.3%. A higher case–fatality rate may occur in adults over 50 years of age.

Type of illness	**Amoebiasis (amoebic dysentery)**
ICD code	ICD-9: 006 ICD-10: A06
Etiological agent	**Protozoa**: *Entamoeba histolytica*.
Characteristics of the agent	An amoeboid protozoan that is an aerotolerant anaerobe. It survives in the environment in an encysted form. Cysts remain viable and infective for several days in faeces and may survive in soil for at least 8 days at 28–34 °C, and for more than 1 month at 10 °C. Relatively resistant to chlorine.
Incubation period	2–4 weeks, but may range from a few days to several months.
Symptoms	Severe bloody diarrhoea, stomach pains, fever and vomiting. Most infections remains symptomless.
Sequelae	Liver abscess.
Duration	Weeks–months.
Reservoir/source	Mainly humans, but also dogs and rats. The organism is also found in nightsoil, and sewage irrigation.
Mode of transmission and example of foods involved in outbreaks	Transmission occurs mainly through the ingestion of faecally contaminated food and water containing cysts. Cysts are excreted in large numbers (up to 5×10^7 cysts per day) by an infected individual. Illness is spread by the faecal–oral route, person-to-person contact or faecally contaminated food and water. Examples of foods involved include fruit and vegetables, and drinking-water.
Specific control measures	*Industrial*: filtration and disinfection of water supply; hygienic disposal of sewage water, treatment of irrigation water. *Food service establishment/household*: boiling of water, when safe water is not available; thorough washing of fruit and vegetables; thorough cooking of food; good hand hygiene.
Occurrence	Worldwide, particularly in young adults. Estimated rate of occucrrence: very low in industrialized countries: + and very frequent in developing countries with poor sanitation: ++.

Appendix

Type of illness	**Cryptosporidiosis**
ICD code	ICD-9: 136.8 ICD-10: A07.2
Etiological agent	**Protozoa**: *Cryptosporidium parvum*.
Characteristics of the agent	The organism has a complex life cycle that can take place in a single human or animal host. It produces resistant oocysts typically 4–6 m. which are very resistant to the chlorination process, but are killed by conventional cooking procedures.
Incubation period	2–14 days.
Symptoms	Diarrhoea (persistent diarrhoea), nausea, vomiting and abdominal pain sometimes accompanied by an influenza-like illness and fever.
Sequelae	Illness is more serious in the immunocompromised, particularly AIDS patients, and leads to severe nutrient malabsorption and weight loss.
Duration	A few days up to 3 weeks.
Reservoir/source	Humans and wild and domestic animals, e.g. cattle.
Mode of transmission and example of foods involved in outbreaks	Spread through the faecal–oral route, person-to-person contact, or consumption of faecally contaminated food and water. Other routes of transmission include bathing in contaminated swimming pools. Examples of foods involved include raw milk, drinking-water and apple cider.
Specific control measures	*Industrial*: pasteurization/sterilization of milk, filtration and disinfection of water, sanitary disposal of excreta, sewage and wastewater. *Food service establishment/household*: boiling of water when safe water is not available; boiling of milk; thorough cooking of food; good hand hygiene.
Occurrence	Worldwide. Cryptosporidiosis is one of the leading causes of diarrhoeal disease in infants and young children. It constitute 5–15 % of diarrhoeal disease cases in children seen at treatment centres. The estimated rate of occurrence is +++. In industrialized countries, it occurs often in day-care centres. Estimated rate of occurrence: ++.
Other comments	Children under the age of 5 years are more at risk. Immunocompromised individuals, e.g. AIDS patients, may suffer from longer and more severe infection. In AIDS patients, infection may lead to death.

Type of illness	**Giardiasis**
ICD code	ICD-9: 007.1 ICD-10: A.07.1
Etiological agent	**Protozoa**: *Giardia lamblia*.
Characteristics of the agent	This flagellate protozoan has an environmentally resistant cyst stage as well as the vegetative trophozoite stage. Cysts are oval and 7–14 m long. They are resistant to the chlorination process used in most water-treatment systems but are killed by conventional cooking procedures.
Incubation period	4–25 days, usually 7–10 days.
Symptoms	Once ingested, the cysts release the active trophozoite which adheres to the gut wall. Illness is characterized by diarrhoea (which may be chronic and relapsing), abdominal cramps, fatigue, weight loss, anorexia and nausea. It is thought that the symptoms may be caused by a protein toxin.
Sequelae	Cholangitis, dystrophy, joint symptoms, lymphoid hyperplasia.
Duration	Weeks–years.
Reservoir/source	Humans and animals.
Mode of transmission and example of foods involved in outbreaks	*Giardia* cysts are excreted in large numbers by an infected individual. Illness is spread through the faecal–oral route, person-to-person contact or faecally contaminated food and water. Cysts have been isolated from lettuces and fruit such as strawberries. The infection is also associated with drinking-water from surface waters and shallow wells. Examples of foods involved include: water, home-canned salmon and noodle salad.
Specific control measures	*Industrial*: filtration and disinfection of water supply; sanitary disposal of excreta, sewage water, treatment of irrigation water. *Food service establishment/household*: boiling of water, when safe water is not available; thorough washing of fruit and vegetables; thorough cooking of foods; good hand hygiene. *Consumers*: and more specifically campers, should avoid drinking surface water unless it has been boiled or filtered.
Occurrence	Worldwide. In industrialized countries, the estimated rate of occurrence is ++ and in developing countries with poor sanitation +++.
Other comments	Number of asymptomatic carriers is high. Children are affected more frequently than adults. Illness is prolonged and more serious in the immunocompromised, particularly AIDS patients. Tourists are particularly at risk.

Type of illness	**Toxoplasmosis and congenital toxoplasmosis**
ICD code	ICD-9: 130 and 771.2 ICD-10: B58 and P 37.1
Etiological agent	**Protozoa:** *Toxoplasma gondii* (belonging to the family *Sarcocystidae*).
Characteristics of the agent	A coccidian protozoan; infections are often asymptomatic.
Incubation period	5–23 days.
Symptoms	Infections are often asymptomatic or present an acute disease with lymphadenopathy and lymphocytosis persisting for days or weeks.
Sequelae	During pregnancy transplacental infection may cause abortion or stillbirth, chorioretinitis, brain damage. In immunocompromised individuals it may cause cerebritis, chorioretinitis, pneumonia, myocarditis, rash and/or death. Cerebral toxoplasmosis is a particular threat for AIDS patients.
Reservoir/source	Cats and other felines; intermediate hosts are sheep, goats, rodents, pigs, cattle and birds, all of which may carry an infective stage of *T. gondii*, encysted in tissue e.g. muscle or brain, which remains viable for long periods, perhaps the entire life of the animal.
Mode of transmission and example of foods involved in outbreaks	Infections occur through ingestion of oocysts. Children may acquire the infection by playing in sand polluted with cat excreta. Oocysts shed by cats can sporulate and become infective 1–5 days later and may remain infective in water or soil for a year. Infection may also be acquired by eating raw or undercooked meat containing the cysts or food and water contaminated with feline faeces. Transplacental infection may also occur when the infection is acquired during pregnancy. Examples of foods involved include raw or undercooked meat, vegetables and goat's milk.
Specific control measures	*Industrial:* irradiation of meat. *Food service establishments, household:* thorough cooking of meat; careful washing of fruits and vegetables; good personal hygiene — particularly after contact with cats and before food preparation; safe disposal of cat faeces. *Consumers:* particularly, pregnant women if not immune, should be advised to avoid raw or undercooked meat; wash vegetables carefully and wash hands after contact with cats.
Occurrence	Worldwide. Estimated rate of occurrence: + to ++.
Other comments	*T. gondii* cysts remain in the tissue and may reactivate if the immune system becomes compromised, e.g. by cytotoxic or immunosuppressive therapy or in patients with AIDS. In these groups the infection may be fulminant and fatal.

Type of illness	**Anisakiasis**
ICD code	ICD-9: 127.1 ICD-10: B81.0
Etiological agent	**Helminth (nematode/roundworm):** *Anisakis* spp. (larval stage).
Characteristics of the agent	Slender, threadlike parasite measuring 1.5–1.6 cm in length and 0.1 cm in diameter.
Incubation period	A few hours; symptoms related to the intestine a few days or weeks.
Symptoms	The motile larvae burrow into the stomach wall producing acute ulceration and nausea, vomiting and epigastric pain, sometimes with haematemesis. They migrate upward and attach themselves to the oropharynx causing coughing. In the small intestine they cause eosinophilic abscesses.
Reservoir/source	Sea mammals (for *Anisakis* spp. that are parasitic to man).
Mode of transmission and example of foods involved in outbreaks	Consumption of the muscles of some saltwater fish which has been inadequately processed. Examples of foods involved include raw fish dishes (e.g sushi, sashimi, herring, cebiche).
Specific control measures	*Industrial:* irradiation; heat treatment, freezing, candling, cleaning (evisceration) of fish as soon as possible after they are caught (will prevent post-mortem migration of infective larvae from the mesenteries of the fish to muscles). *Food service establishment/household:* cleaning of fish; thorough cooking before consumption; freezing (minus 20°C for 7 days).
Occurrence	Mainly in countries where consumption of raw or inadequately processed fish is common, e.g. Northern Europe, Japan, Latin America. Over 12 000 cases have been reported in Japan. Cases have also been reported in other parts of the world as eating habits change with immigration.
Other comments	Symptoms mimic those of appendicitis.

Type of illness	**Ascariasis**
ICD code	ICD-9: 127.0 ICD-10: B77
Etiological agent	**Helminth (nematode/roundworm):** *Ascaris lumbricoides* (egg with infective larva).
Characteristics of the agent	*Ascaris lumbricoides* is a large roundworm infecting the small intestine. Adult males are 15–31cm x 2–4 mm and females are 20– 40cm x 3–6mm. Eggs undergo embryonation in the soil; after 2–3 weeks at warm temperature they become infective and may remain viable for several months or even years in favourable soils. The larvae emerge from the egg in the duodenum, penetrate the intestinal wall and reach the heart and the lungs in the blood. Larvae grow and develop in the lungs; 9–10 days after infection they break out of the pulmonary capillaries into the alveoli and migrate through the bronchial tubes and trachea of the pharynx where they are swallowed and reach the intestine 14–20 days after infection. In the intestine they develop into adults and begin laying eggs 40–60 days after ingestion of the embryonated eggs. The life cycle is complete after 8 weeks.
Incubation period	First appearance of eggs in stools is 60–70 days. In larval ascariasis, symptoms occur 4–16 days after infection.
Symptoms	Gastrointestinal discomfort, colic and vomiting, fever; observation of live worms in stools. Some patients may have pulmonary symptoms or neurological disorders during migration of the larvae. However there are generally few or no symptoms.
Sequelae	A heavy worm infestation may cause nutritional deficiency; other complications, sometimes fatal, include obstruction of the bowel by a bolus of worms (observed particularly in children), obstruction of bile or pancreatic duct.
Reservoir/source	Humans; soil and vegetation on which faecal matter containing eggs has been deposited.
Mode of transmission and example of foods involved in outbreaks	Ingestion of infective eggs from soil contaminated with human faeces or contaminated vegetables and water.
Specific control measures	Use of toilet facilities; safe excreta disposal; protection of food from dirt and soil; thorough washing of produce. Food dropped on the floor should not be eaten without washing or cooking, particularly in endemic areas.
Occurrence	Worldwide. There is a high prevalence (exceeding 50%) in moist and tropical countries. Estimated rate of occurrence: + to +++ depending on the region.
Other comments	In endemic areas the highest prevalence is among children aged 3–8 years.

Type of illness	**Trichinellosis (trichiniasis, trichinosis)**
ICD code	ICD-9: 124 ICD-10: B75
Etiological agent	**Helminth (nematode/roundworm):** *Trichinella spiralis* (larvae in infected muscle).
Characteristics of the agent	White intestinal worm, visible to the naked eye. The transmissible form of this parasite is a larval cyst approximately 0.4 mm x 0.25 mm which occurs in pork muscle. In the initial phase of trichinellosis, the larvae ingested with the meat develop rapidly into adults in the epithelium of the intestine. Female worms produce larvae which penetrate the lymphatics or venules and are disseminated via the blood throughout the body. The larvae become encapsulated in the skeletal muscle.
Incubation period	Initial phase: a few days. Systemic symptoms: 8–21 days.
Symptoms	Symptoms range from inapparent infection to fulminating and fatal disease, depending on the number of larvae ingested. Symptoms during the initial invasion are nausea, vomiting, diarrhoea and fever. During the phase of parasite dissemination to the tissues, there may be rheumatic manifestations, muscle soreness and pain together with oedema of the upper eyelids, sometimes followed by subconjunctival, subungual and retinal haemorrhages, pain and photophobia. Thirst, profuse sweating, chills, weakness, prostration and rapidly increasing eosinophilia may follow shortly after the ocular symptoms.
Sequelae	Cardiac and neurological complications may appear in weeks 3–6; in the most severe cases death due to myocardial failure may occur.
Duration	2 weeks to 2–3 months.
Reservoir/source	Pigs, dogs, cats, rats, horses and other mammals of man's domestic environment.
Mode of transmission and example of foods involved in outbreaks	Ingestion of raw or undercooked meat (pork, horse) containing the encysted larvae. Examples of foods involved include pork, horse, wild boar, game.
Specific control measures	*Industrial:* irradiation of meat, freezing, heating and curing. *Food service establishment/household:* thorough cooking of meat, freezing (minus 15 °C for 30 days). Additionally, hunters should thoroughly cook all game.
Occurrence	Worldwide, with predominance in countries where pork or game is eaten. Estimated rate of occurrence varies from + to ++ in high prevalence areas.

Type of illness	**Taeniasis**: *Taenia solium* taeniasis and cysticercosis *Taenia saginata* taeniasis
ICD code	ICD-9: 123.0 (*Taenia solium* taeniasis); 123.2 (*Taenia saginata* taeniasis); 123.1 (cysticercosis) ICD-10: B68.0 (*Taenia solium* taeniasis); B68.1 (*Taenia saginata* taeniasis), B69 (cysticercosis)
Etiological agent	**Helminth (cestode/tapeworm)**: *Taenia solium* and *Cysticercus cellulosae* (larvae of *T. solium*) and *Taenia saginata* and *Cysticercus bovis* (larvae of *T. saginata*).
Characteristics of the agent	*T. solium* causes both intestinal infection with adult worms as well as somatic infection with the eggs. The adult worm comprises a scolex 1 mm in diameter, armed with two rows of hooks and four suckers. The strobila ranges in length from 1.8–4 m. *T. saginata* causes only intestinal infection with adult worms. The adult worm comprises a scolex 1–2 mm in diameter, equipped with four suckers, a neck, and a strobila that ranges in length from 35 mm to 6 m.
Incubation period	Symptoms of cysticercosis appear from a few days to over 10 years. Eggs appear in the stools 8–12 weeks after infection with *T. solium*, and 10–14 weeks after infection with *T. saginata*.
Symptoms	Nervousness, insomnia, anorexia, weight loss, abdominal pain and digestive disturbance. Cysticercosis may cause epileptiform seizures, signs of intracranial hypertension or psychiatric disturbance. Cysticercosis may be fatal.
Sequelae	Cysticercosis may affect the central nervous system. When eggs or proglottides of *T. solium* are swallowed, the eggs hatch in the small intestine and the larvae migrate to subcutaneous tissue, striated muscles, and other tissues and vital organs of the body where they form cysts. Severe health consequences occur when the larvae localize in the eye, central nervous system or heart.
Reservoir/source	Humans; pigs and cattle are the intermediate host for *T. solium* and *T. saginata*.
Mode of transmission and example of foods involved in outbreaks	Taeniasis is caused by consumption of raw or undercooked beef (*Taenia saginata*) or pork (*Taenia solium*) containing cysticerci. Gravid proglottides of the parasite are excreted in faeces. Eggs within the segments are infective. Cattle ingest the eggs deposited on pasture and pigs ingest those deposited on soil. When viable eggs are ingested by cattle or pigs they develop into cysticerci in the muscle. Cysticercosis is caused by ingestion of *T. solium* eggs by the faecal–oral route, person-to-person contact, autoinfection (unwashed hands) or consumption of contaminated food e.g. vegetables.
Specific control measures	*Industrial*: prevention of faecal contamination of soil, water, human and animal food through safe disposal of sewage; avoidance of sewage water for irrigation use. Irradiation, heat treatment, and freezing kills the cysticerci. *Food service establishment/household*: thorough cooking of meat. *Other*: early diagnosis and treatment to prevent cysticercosis.
Occurrence	Worldwide. Most common in Africa, Latin America, eastern Europe, and south-east Asia. Estimated rate of occurrence varies from + to ++ in high prevalence areas.
Other comments	*T. saginata* eggs are infective only in cattle, *T. solium* eggs are infective in pigs and humans. Eggs of both species are disseminated in the environment as long as the worm remains in the intestine, sometimes for more than 30 years; eggs may remain viable in the environment for months.

Type of illness	**Clonorchiasis**
ICD code	ICD-9: 121.1 ICD-10: B66.1
Etiological agent	**Helminth (trematode/flatworm):** *Clonorchis sinensis*, also known as Chinese or oriental liver fluke.
Characteristics of the agent	This is a flattened worm, 10–25 mm long, 3–5 mm wide and usually spatula shaped. It is yellow-brown, owing to bile staining; has an oral and a ventral sucker and is a hermaphrodite. Eggs measure 20–30 μm x 15–17 μm; they are operculate and one of the smallest trematode eggs to occur in man.
Incubation period	Unpredictable: varies with the number of worms present. Symptoms begin with the entry of immature flukes into the biliary system, within one month after encysted larvae (metacercarie) are ingested.
Symptoms	Gradual onset of discomfort in the right upper quadrant, anorexia, indigestion, abdominal pain or distension and irregular bowel movement. Patients who are heavily infected experience weakness, weight loss, epigastric discomfort, abdominal fullness, diarrhoea, anaemia, oedema. In the later stages, jaundice, portal hypertension, ascites and upper gastointestinal bleeding occur.
Sequelae	The liver (predominantly the left lobe) is enlarged. The spleen can be palpated in only a small percentage of infected cases. Recurrent pyogenic cholangitis is a serious complication of clonorchiasis. The pancreas may be involved in severe cases of *C. sinensis* infection. The pathology of pancreatic clonorchiasis is similar to that of hepatic lesion, namely adenomatous hyperplasia of the ductal epithelium. When acute pancreatitis occurs, inflammation is present. Cholangiocarcinoma is also associated with clonorchiasis. Repeated or heavy infection during childhood has been reported to cause dwarfism with retarded sexual development.
Reservoir/source	Snails are the first intermediate host. Some 40 species of river fish serve as the second intermediate host. Humans, dogs, cats and many other species of fish-eating mammals are definitive hosts.
Mode of transmission and example of foods involved in outbreaks	People are infected by eating raw or under-processed freshwater fish containing encysted larvae (metacercariae). During digestion, the larvae are freed from the cysts and migrate via the common bile duct to biliary radicles. Eggs deposited in the bile passages are evacuated in faeces. Eggs in faeces contain fully developed miracidia; when ingested by a susceptible operculate snail, they hatch in its intestine, penetrate the tissues and asexually generate larvae (cercariae) that migrate into the water. On contact with a second intermediate host, the cercariae penetrate the host and encyst, usually in muscle, occasionally on the underside of scales. The complete life cycle from person to snail to fish to person requires at least 3 months.
Specific control measures	*Industrial:* Safe disposal of excreta and sewage/wastewater to prevent contamination of rivers; treatment of wastewater used for aquaculture; irradiation of freshwater fish; freezing; heat treatment, e.g. canning. *Food service establishment/household:* thorough cooking of freshwater fish. *Consumers* should avoid consumption of raw or undercooked freshwater fish. *Other:* control of snails with molluscicides where feasible; drug treatment of the population to reduce the reservoir of infection; elimination of stray dogs and cats.
Occurrence	Endemic in Western Pacific areas: China, Hong Kong, Japan, Malaysia, Republic of Korea, Singapore, Thailand, Viet Nam. Estimated rate of occurrence: ++/+++. In Europe: eastern part of Russian Federation (Estimated rate of occurrence: ++).
Other comments	About one-third of chronic infections are asymptomatic.

Type of illness	**Fascioliasis**
ICD code	ICD-9: 121.3 ICD-10: B66.3
Etiological agent	**Helminth (trematode/flatworm/liver fluke):** *Fasciola hepatica* and *Fasciola gigantica*.
Characteristics of the agent	*Fasciola hepatica*: large fluke (23–30 mm x 15 mm), pale grey in colour with dark borders, leaf-shaped with a distinct cephalic cone at the anterior end. Eggs are usually 130–150 µm x 63–90 µm. They have an inconspicuous operculum, are non-embryonated, and often have a shell irregularity at the abopercular end. *Fasciola gigantica* is bigger and may attein a length of 75 mm.
Incubation period	4–6 weeks.
Symptoms	Fever, sweating, abdominal pain, dizziness, cough, bronchial asthma, urticaria. In children, the acute infection is accompanied by severe clinical manifestations, including right upper quadrant pain or generalized abdominal pain, fever and anaemia, and can be fatal. Ectopic infections are common in man.
Sequelae	Necrotic lesions, inflammatory, adenomatous and fibrotic changes in the bile duct, biliary stasis, atrophy of the liver and periportal cirrhosis, cholecystitis and cholelithiasis.
Reservoir/source	Snails are the intermediate host; sheep, cattle and humans are the definitive host.
Mode of transmission and example of foods involved in outbreaks	Infection in human is associated with the consumption of uncultivated raw watercress (*Nasturtium officinale*) and other salad plants, such as dandelions, bearing metacercariae. After ingestion, the larvae are released from the cyst envelopes into the duodenum, pass through the intestinal wall to the abdominal cavity, enter the liver and after development enter the bile ducts and begin laying non-embryonated eggs 3–4 months after initial exposure. The eggs are carried by the bile into the intestine, and evacuated with the faeces. The eggs mature and the miracidia emerge from the eggs to the water in a few weeks. The miracidia penetrate the snail (intermediate host), and turn into sporocysts and in about 3 weeks produce rediae which, in turn, produce cercariae. The cercariae may begin to emerge from the snails in six weeks under favourable conditions. After leaving the snail, the cercariae swim in the water and cyst on vegetation, turning into metacercariae which can survive for a long time in a wet environment. The life cycle is then complete.
Specific control measures	*Industrial:* safe disposal of excreta and sewage/wastewater; drug treatment of livestock against the parasite; prevention of animal access to commercial watercress beds and control of water used to irrigate the beds. *Food service establishment/household:* thorough cooking of food. *Consumers* should avoid consumption of raw watercress. *Others:* control of snails with molluscicides where feasible; drug treatment of the population to reduce the reservoir of infection.
Occurrence	Africa, e.g. Egypt, Ethiopia; Americas, e.g. Bolivia, Ecuador, Peru; Asia, e.g. China; Islamic Republic of Iran; Europe: France, Portugal, Spain. The estimated rate of occurrence varies, depending on the country, from ++ to +++.

Type of illness	**Opisthorchiasis**
ICD code	ICD-9: 121.0 ICD-10: B66.0
Etiological agent	**Helminth (trematode/flatworm/liver fluke)**: *Opisthorchis viverrini* and *Opisthorchis felineus*.
Characteristics of the agent	Morphological features resemble that of *Clonorchis sinensis*. The worm lives in the intrahepatic bile ducts and pancreas and has been also found in the lungs. It measures 8–11 mm x 1.5–2 mm. Eggs measure 30 µm x 12 µm and are slenderer than the *C. sinensis* eggs.
Incubation period	*Opisthorchis felineus*: 2–4 weeks, very occasionally 1 week.
Symptoms	Fever, abdominal pain, dizziness, urticaria. Chronic cases may lead to diarrhoea, flatulence, fatty food intolerance, epigastric and right upper quadrant pain, jaundice, fever, hepatomegaly, lassitude, anorexia, and in some cases emaciation and oedema.
Sequelae	Cholecystitis, cholangitis, liver abscess and gallstones. Cholangiocarcinoma is associated with *O. viverrini* infection and perhaps also with *O. felineus*.
Reservoir/source	The first intermediate host is the freshwater snail; several fish species act as second intermediate host. Humans, dogs, cats, and other mammals that eat fish or fish waste are definitive hosts.
Mode of transmission and example of foods involved in outbreaks	Humans are infected by consumption of raw or under-processed freshwater fish. The life cycle of *Opisthorchis* is similar to that of *C. sinesis*.
Specific control measures	*Industrial*: safe disposal of excreta and sewage/wastewater; treatment of wastewater used for aquaculture; irradiation of freshwater fish; freezing; heat treatment e.g. canning. *Food service establishment/household*: thorough cooking of freshwater fish. Consumers should avoid consumption of raw or undercooked freshwater fish. *Others* control of snails with molluscicides where feasible; drug treatment of the population to reduce the reservoir of infection; elimination of stray dogs and cats.
Occurrence	*Opisthorchis viverrini*: Cambodia, Lao Peoples Democratic Republic, Thailand. *Opisthorchis felineus*: Europe: Baltic states, eastern Germany, Kazakhstan, Poland, the Russian Federation, Ukraine; Asia: India, Japan, Thailand. In European countries the estimated rate of occurrence is ++ and in Asian countries, the estimated rate of occurrence is +++.

Type of illness	Paragonimiasis
ICD code	ICD-9: 121.2 ICD-10: B66.4
Etiological agent	**Helminth (trematode/flatworm/lung fluke)**: *Paragonimus westermani* (metacercariae).
Characteristics of the agent	This is a reddish brown hermaphrodite which measures 10–12 mm in length and 5–7 mm in width (adult). The shape varies from linear to spherical. Eggs usually measure 80–120 µm, are golden brown in color, thick-shelled, non-embryonated in faeces or in sputum and have a prominent operculum. The shell is thickened at the abopercular end.
Incubation period	Acute stage: a few days to several weeks. Chronic stage: pulmonary symptoms begin at around 3 months.
Symptoms	The early stages are usually asymptomatic. However, heavily infected patients may experience fever, fatigue, generalized myalgia and abdominal pain with eosinophilia.
Sequelae	Pleuropulmonary paragonimiasis (pulmonary lesion): chronic coughing, thoracic pain, blood-stained viscous sputum. Systemic symptoms of fatigue, fever, myalgia, chest pain and dyspnoea. Severe infections produce tuberculosis-like symptoms. Ectopic paragonimiasis (extrapulmonary lesion): migration of the worm through the brain can cause cerebral haemorrhage, oedema or meningitis. Severe headache, mental confusion, seizure, hemiparesis, hypaesthesia, blurred vision, diplopia, homonymous hemianopsia and meningismus may occur. Abdominal paragonimiasis: results in abdominal pain, and there may be diarrhoea with blood and mucus when the intestinal mucosa is ulcerated.
Reservoir/source	Fresh-water snails are the first intermediate host; crabs and crayfish are second intermediate hosts. Humans, dogs, pigs and other wild and domestic animals are definitive hosts.
Mode of transmission and example of foods involved in outbreaks	The definitive hosts are infected through consumption of raw, inadequately cooked or otherwise under-processed freshwater crustaceans (crabs and crayfish) which contain the metacercariae, or the contamination of other food items, hands and cooking utensils by the metacercariae released from infected crabs during food preparation. Following ingestion, the metacercariae *(P. westermani)* in the infected crustaceans excyst in the duodenum of the host and the larvae penetrate the intestinal wall and migrate beneath the peritoneum where they remain for 5–7 days. Over a period of about 2–3 weeks following infection, the immature worms penetrate the diaphragm, enter the pleural cavity and then move into the lung parenchyma where they mature. At this stage, eggs may be present in the sputum without the host showing any symptoms. During the intial stage of lung infection, the adult worms migrate through the tissues and cause focal haemorrhagic pneumonia. After 12 weeks, the worms in the lung parenchyma typically provoke a granulomatus reaction that gradually proceeds to development of fibrotic encapsulation. Extrapulmonary lesions are caused by worms that reach and develop in ectopic foci.
Specific control measures	*Industrial:* safe disposal of excreta and sewage/wastewater to prevent contamination of rivers. *Food service establishment/household:* thorough cooking of food, i.e. crabs and crayfish, and hygienic handling of these foods. *Consumers* should avoid consumption of raw or undercooked or under-processed crabs and crayfish. *Others:* control of snails with molluscicides where feasible; drug treatment of the population to reduce the reservoir of infection; elimination of stray dogs and cats.
Occurrence	Africa, e.g. Cameroon, Nigeria; Americas, e.g. Ecuador, Peru; Asia, e.g. China, Japan, Lao People's Democratic Republic, Philippines, Republic of Korea, Thailand. Estimated rate of occurrence in these countries is +++.

Appendix 2

WHO's Ten Golden Rules for Safe Food Preparation

The following rules have been drawn up by WHO to provide guidance on safe food preparation in the home. They should be adapted, as appropriate, to local conditions.

1. Choose foods processed for safety

While many foods, such as fruits and vegetables, are best in their natural state, others simply are not safe unless they have been processed. For example, always buy pasteurized as opposed to raw milk and, if you have the choice, select fresh or frozen poultry treated with ionizing radiation. When shopping, keep in mind that food processing was invented to improve safety as well as to prolong shelf-life. Certain foods eaten raw, such as lettuce, need thorough washing.

2. Cook food thoroughly

Many raw foods, most notably poultry, meats, eggs and unpasteurized milk, may be contaminated with disease-causing organisms. Thorough cooking will kill the pathogens, but remember that the temperature of all parts of the food must reach at least 70 °C. If cooked chicken is still raw near the bone, put it back in the oven until it's done — all the way through. Frozen meat, fish, and poultry must be thoroughly thawed before cooking.

3. Eat cooked foods immediately

When cooked foods cool to room temperature, microbes begin to proliferate. The longer the wait, the greater the risk. To be on the safe side, eat cooked foods just as soon as they come off the heat.

4. Store cooked foods carefully

If you must prepare foods in advance or want to keep leftovers, be sure to store them under either hot (near or above 60 °C) or cool (near or below 10 °C) conditions. This rule is of vital importance if you plan to store foods for more than four or five hours. Foods for infants should preferably not be stored at all. A common error, responsible for countless cases of foodborne disease, is putting too large a quantity of warm food in the refrigerator. In an overburdened refrigerator, cooked foods cannot cool to the core as quickly as they must. When the centre of food remains warm (above 10 °C) too long, microbes thrive, quickly proliferating to disease-causing levels.

5. Reheat cooked foods thoroughly

This is your best protection against microbes that may have developed during storage (proper storage slows down microbial growth but does not kill the organisms). Once again, thorough reheating means that all parts of the food must reach at least 70 °C.

6. Avoid contact between raw foods and cooked foods

Safely cooked food can become contaminated through even the slightest contact with raw food. This cross-contamination can be direct, as when raw poultry meat comes into contact with cooked foods. It can also be more subtle. For example, don't prepare a raw chicken and then use the same unwashed cutting board and knife to carve the cooked bird. Doing so can reintroduce the disease-causing organisms.

7. Wash hands repeatedly

Wash hands thoroughly before you start preparing food and after every interruption — especially if you have to change the baby or have been to the toilet. After preparing raw foods such as fish, meat, or poultry, wash again before you start handling other foods. And if you have an infection on your hand, be sure to bandage or cover it before preparing food. Remember, too, that household pets — dogs, cats, birds, and especially turtles — often harbour dangerous pathogens that can pass from your hands into food.

8. Keep all kitchen surfaces meticulously clean

Since foods are so easily contaminated, any surface used for food preparation must be kept absolutely clean. Think of every food scrap, crumb or spot as a potential reservoir of germs. Cloths that come into contact with dishes and utensils should be changed frequently and boiled before re-use. Separate cloths for cleaning the floors also require frequent washing.

9. Protect food from insects, rodents, and other animals

Animals frequently carry pathogenic microorganisms which cause foodborne disease. Storing foods in closed containers is your best protection.

10. Use safe water

Safe water is just as important for food preparation as for drinking. If you have any doubts about the water supply, boil water before adding it to food or making ice for drinks. Be especially careful with any water used to prepare an infant's meal.

Appendix 3

The Hazard Analysis and Critical Control Point system (HACCP)[1]

HACCP is an approach that identifies specific hazards[2] and measures for their control. Its full implementation consists of seven principles.

1. Conduct a hazard analysis
This identifies and evaluates the potential hazards that may reasonably be expected to occur at each step of food production from growth, harvesting or slaughter, processing and manufacturing, distribution, and preparation through to final consumption. At each stage, the likelihood of occurrence of hazards and the severity of their adverse health effects are assessed, and measures for their control are identified.

2. Determine critical control points
These are steps at which control can be applied and is essential to prevent, eliminate or reduce a hazard to an acceptable level.

3. Establish critical limits
Critical limits are criteria which separate acceptability from unacceptability. A critical limit may be, for example, a particular temperature, a temperature–time combination, a pH value, or a salt content that is known to control a hazard if it is achieved. For example, a pH of 4.5 or below is known to prevent the growth of *Clostridium botulinum*, this would therefore be a critical limit that, if achieved, would ensure control of that hazard.

4. Establish monitoring systems
An essential part of HACCP is to monitor control parameters (e.g. time-temperature, pH) at critical control points in order to ensure that control of hazards is being exercised and critical limits are observed. In commercial food processing/production this means the introduction of a schedule of testing or observation.

5. Establish corrective actions
If monitoring indicates that a critical limit has not been observed, it is necessary to know what action to take to correct the situation and to deal with the food that was produced while the critical control point was not under control. For example, a food might have to be reheated.

---

[1] The description of the HACCP system presented here is based on an adaptation of the Codex Alimentarius Commission's text on Hazard Analysis and Critical Control Point System and Guidelines for its Application. Codex Alimentarius Commission. Food Hygiene Basic Texts. Rome, Secretariat of the Joint FAO/WHO Food Standards Programme, 1997.

[2] A hazard is a biological, chemical or physical agent in, or condition of, food with the potential to cause an adverse health effect.

6. Establish verification procedures
Verification includes supplementary tests and procedures which will confirm that the HACCP system is working effectively. It could also indicate that an HACCP plan requires modification.

7. Establish documentation and record keeping
This should cover all documentation and records appropriate to the HACCP scheme, such as details of the hazard analysis, CCP and critical limit determination and results from monitoring and verification. Documentation and record keeping should be appropriate to the nature of the operation.

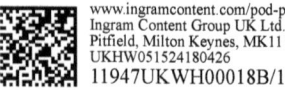
www.ingramcontent.com/pod-product-compliance
Ingram Content Group UK Ltd.
Pitfield, Milton Keynes, MK11 3LW, UK
UKHW051524180426
11947UKWH00018B/1557